everyday arthritis SOLUTIONS

STOP ARTHRITIS FROM STOPPING YOU

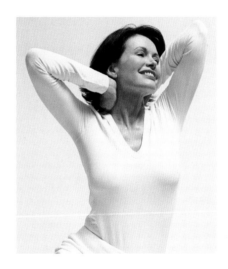

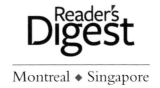

Reader's Digest

Montreal ◆ Singapore

Project Staff

Editors: **Jesse Corbeil, Nancy Shuker**

Writer: **Richard Laliberte**

Consultants: **Virginia Byers Kraus, MD PhD, Daniel S. Rooks, PhD**

Copy Editor: **Jeanette Gingold**

Proofreader: **J.D. Gravenor**

Design: **Andrée Payette, Michele Laseau**

Manager, English Book Editorial: **Pamela Johnson**

Production Manager: **Gordon Howlett**

Production Coordinator: **Gillian Sylvain**

Photographer: **Jill Wachter**

Photo Art Direction: **Marian Purcell-Solid Design**

Indexer: **Patricia Buchanan**

Reader's Digest Association (Canada) ULC

Vice-President, Book Editorial:
Robert Goyette

Reader's Digest Health Publishing

Editor-in-Chief and Publishing Director:
Neil Wertheimer

Reader's Digest Association, Inc.

President and Chief Executive Officer:
Mary Berner

Note to Readers

The information in this book should not be substituted for, or used to alter, any medical treatment or therapy without your doctor's advice.

Library and Archives Canada Cataloguing in Publication

Everyday arthritis solutions : stop arthritis from stopping you / the editors of Reader's Digest. -- 1st Canadian ed.

Includes index.
ISBN 978-1-55475-014-6

1. Arthritis--Treatment--Popular works.
2. Arthritis--Alternative treatment--Popular works.
I. Reader's Digest Association (Canada)

RC933.E84 2009   616.7'2206   C2009-900224-8

Address any comments about *Everyday Arthritis Solutions* to:

The Reader's Digest Association (Canada), ULC

Book Editor

1100 René-Lévesque Blvd. West

Montreal QC H3B 5H5

To order copies of *Everyday Arthritis Solutions*, call 1-800-465-0780

Visit our website at **rd.ca**

Printed in China

09 10 11 12 / 5 4 3 2 1

introduction

You want to move freely every day. You want to have energy every day. You want to eat well every day. You want life to be filled with potential every day.

What's stopping you? We hope you didn't say "arthritis." But if you did, we are here to convince you otherwise. For as painful and debilitating as arthritis can be, there are effective solutions emerging that will give you far greater mobility and far less pain than you might expect.

Not long ago, a diagnosis of arthritis typically came with a recommendation for painkillers, rest and resignation. But research has proved this to be a misguided prescription. Today we know that:

- movement and exercise are among the very best remedies for arthritis;

- certain foods are rich in nutrients that can help your suffering joints;

- certain supplements can significantly improve joint health and healing;

- a positive outlook and an active lifestyle will go a long way toward minimizing the impact of arthritis.

What's terrific about these findings is that they put your life back under your control. Yes, you need a doctor to prescribe a medicine, but only you can decide to take a walk through your neighbourhood, or to have shrimp for supper rather than steak—and yes, shrimp is an arthritis "superfood"!

Everyday Arthritis Solutions brings you the newest arthritis wisdom and most effective ways to manage your condition. There are a lot of pages inside filled with exercise photos, but don't be fooled into thinking this is merely a fitness book. Look closely and you'll discover hundreds of clever hints and tips for managing everyday life with arthritis—the best foods to eat, the right supplements to take, even the best meals to cook.

And then there are the exercises. Please don't be intimidated. We believe we have put together one of the most usable, comfortable sets of movements possible for people with arthritis. Sample them like recipes in a cookbook, and then turn to Part Four to learn how to put them together into 5- to 15-minute routines for your particular needs and abilities. Current research shows that there is nothing better you can do for arthritis than to strengthen joint muscles and to keep on moving. Here, for the first time, is the ultimate set of exercises for exactly your needs.

Indeed, we believe we have put together the most thorough guide to date for self-managing arthritis. The doctors and writers who worked on this book are the very best in their respective fields, and the results show. So take control of your condition. Give these exercises, tips, supplements, and recipes a try, and we promise you, *every* day will be a best day.

The Editors of Reader's Digest

table of contents

introduction *3*

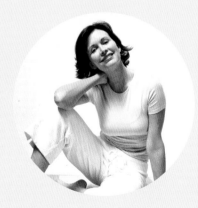

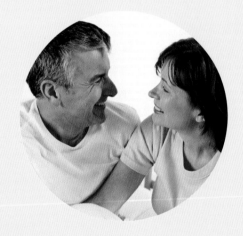

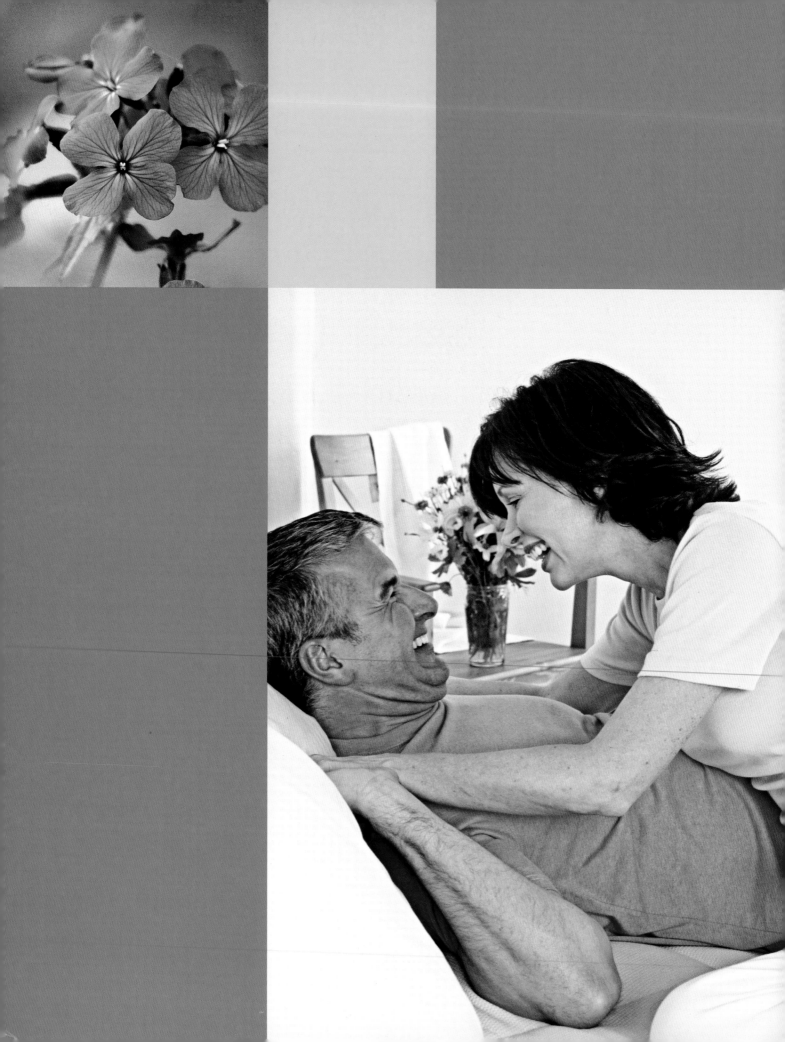

know your arthritis

Knowing how a healthy body works, and

understanding what goes wrong when arthritis strikes, can

help you get the upper hand on treatment and pain relief.

Knowledge and a good attitude will also transform you into

a motivated, full-time partner in your own health care.

The result? Simple: increased mobility and

independence, and a better quality of life.

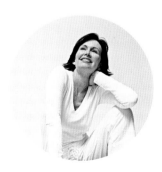

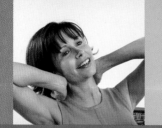
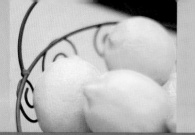

knowledge is power

Many people suffering from arthritis are caught up in a devastating cycle of pain, stress and depression. But taking on an active role in managing your pain can help break that vicious cycle. Boning up on your condition is an excellent way to help take the fear out of the arthritis equation—knowing what's going on with your body can bring a much-needed sense of calm and enable you to make clear-headed decisions.

An Equal-Opportunity Condition

The word "arthritis" does not refer to one simple condition; it encompasses some 127 different diseases. So when someone says that they have arthritis, the logical response is, "What kind?" Arthritis, in its many forms, can strike all ages and both sexes. Some forms—rheumatoid arthritis, fibromyalgia and lupus—are more prevalent among women; gout and ankylosing spondylitis are more common in men.

Indeed, arthritis has many faces. It may affect only one joint or it may involve an immune attack against many of them. One person may experience excruciating pain and fatigue while another experiences only mild aches. Your symptoms may fluctuate between great pain and periods of quiescence while a friend's symptoms may remain stable for years. Some forms of the disease are caused by metabolic disorders, while others are genetically determined and still others may result from environmental factors—what we do or don't eat, for example.

Take action to fight arthritis. A generation ago, the words "arthritis" and "action" were seldom spoken in the same sentence. Arthritis was thought of as a chronic, debilitating disease that slowed you down and ultimately left you hobbled. Action was what arthritis prevented. Or so it was thought.

We live in a more enlightened time. Not that arthritis is less serious or pervasive than it ever was. It remains a leading cause of disability in the country, and if you have it, you can take grim comfort in the fact that at least 4.5 million other Canadians share some form of your pain. No one has yet found a way to cure arthritis. But passively watching as your function and mobility erode is no longer an acceptable course of action. In fact, action is not only possible with arthritis, it's the key to reducing pain and continuing to lead a productive, vigorous life.

Action against arthritis takes two forms. The first is fighting the disease itself with all the medical, physical and psychological weapons at your disposal. The second is simply living life to the fullest—staying active, moving your body, working your joints and stretching your muscles. Living fully also means enjoying a robust and satisfying diet while controlling your weight and getting adequate amounts of the specific nutrients thought to help ease arthritis symptoms. In short, taking action by living well promises to let you be even more active—and enjoy a better quality of life.

Research pioneered at Stanford University shows that by using what scientists call arthritis self-management—in which exercise and healthy nutrition play a central role—you can tame arthritis pain, maintain function, and even make remarkable improvements. No more relying on doctors to tell you what to do. The self-management view puts you squarely in charge, instead enlisting doctors and other caregivers to support you with treatment and advice. Studies find that nonmedical habits, attitudes and activities that you alone control often make the biggest difference in easing pain and enjoying life. Consider: Follow-up research has found that even 20 months after learning more about exercise, diet and other subjects as part of self-help courses, arthritis sufferers on average:

- Reduced pain by 20 percent
- Eased depression by 14 percent
- Cut doctor visits by 35 percent

What's more, patients largely continued reaping these benefits as long as four years after first learning to call their own shots.

This book is chock full of detailed information and advice aimed at helping you to harness the power of exercise and good nutrition to beat back arthritis. These elements fit into a bigger action plan built on a variety of strategies.

Elements of a good action plan include becoming an informed manager of your own health, getting the right medical assistance, controlling your pain, restoring and maintaining joint functionality, and managing your weight. These strategies, in conjunction with a can-do attitude and a goal-oriented approach will help get you back on your feet. Later chapters will go into more detail, laying out the building blocks for an effective arthritis action plan, from excercise routines to methods for dealing with flare-ups and recipes for delicious, arthritis-busting meals.

Information is power. Whereas later chapters will explore treatments in depth (exercise, drugs and nutrition, as well as stress-reduction techniques and alternative approaches that can help you overcome your arthritis problem), this chapter provides a rundown of the most common types of arthritis. In each case, we describe the condition and its causes, as well as the progression of symptoms. We also discuss how each type of arthritis is diagnosed, what you should do after a positive diagnosis and the most promising treatments. We also take a look at nutritional suplements and complementary treatments.

We begin, however, with a primer on the anatomy of a joint—ground zero for virtually every type of arthritis.

THE FEMININE SIDE OF ARTHRITIS

According to The Arthritis Society, some 2.9 million Canadian women are believed to suffer from some type of arthritis and the number is expected to reach 3.9 million by 2026—nearly twice the number of men. Theories abound, ranging from the belief that women's weaker cartilage and tendons are the cause, right up to a link with estrogen. All are unproven, but the statistics are undeniable. For example:

Osteoarthritis affects 3,000,000 (or one in 10) Canadians, with twice as many women suffering from the disease as men, according to the Arthritis Community Research & Evaluation Unit. Most OA sufferers develop the condition after 45, but it can strike at any age.

Rheumatoid Arthritis affects 300,000 (or one in 100) Canadians and affects three times as many women as men. Most RA sufferers develop the condition between the ages of 25 and 30, but it can strike anyone, from babies to the elderly.

Lupus (systemic lupus erythematosus, AKA SLE) affects 15,000 (or one in 2,000) Canadians. Women develop lupus eight to 10 times as often as men, usually between the ages of 15 and 45. But the disease can strike any time from babyhood to old age.

Polymyalgia affects 300,000 (or one in 100) Canadians and three times as many women as men. Most develop the disease between 25 and 50, but it can strike any time.

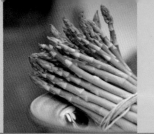
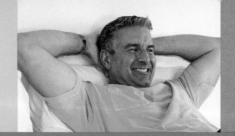

bones and joints 101

Bones are connected to each other at joints. The body's joints can be grouped into three classes based on the amount of movement they allow: fixed joints, slightly movable joints and freely movable joints.

Fixed joints. These joints allow no movement whatever. Examples of fixed joints include those separating the bones of the pelvis, which bend only during delivery to ease the baby's movement down the birth canal and the joints (known as sutures) between the bones of the skull.

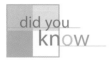

By age 65, more than half of all people have X-ray evidence of osteoarthritis in at least one joint.

Slightly movable joints. These joints allow a limited amount of motion. For example, the bones of the spinal column are held together by tough pads of fibrocartilage. These so-called intervertebral joints secure the bones tightly while still providing the flexibility to let you bend and stretch.

Freely movable (or synovial) joints. These are the joints that usually leap to mind when we think of arthritis. Examples are the hips, knees, elbows, fingers and—most mobile of all—the shoulder joint, whose ball-and-socket structure enables you to move your arm in a complete circle.

➡ BONING UP: The human skeleton

contains more than 200 bones, which are

connected by almost 150 joints.

Joint capsule

The bones of the joint are covered by a tough, fibrous covering called the joint capsule. The capsule's outer layer is made of interwoven bands of collagen fibres, which provide the joint capsule with strength and flexibility.

Synovial membrane

This is a delicate layer of tissue that lines the joint capsule's inner surface, producing and releasing synovial fluid. This clear, sticky fluid is 95 percent water, has the consistency of egg white (synovia means "like egg white") and helps nourish and lubricate the cartilage and bones within the joint capsule. Aided by the synovial fluid, the cartilage-tipped bones in a healthy joint glide over each other smoothly, creating even less friction than ice sliding on ice.

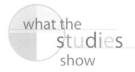

what the studies show

Exercises that protect and strengthen the muscles, tendons, and ligaments that surround a joint can minimize pain and stiffness within the joint itself.

Ligaments

These strong, flexible bands of connective tissue are made of collagen fibres, and help to stabilize a joint by binding together the bones within it. Most ligaments lack elasticity, but some stretch a little to allow the bones that they connect to separate slightly. Others prevent the joint from moving a certain way. If you dislocate a joint, it is best to get it corrected immediately, as ligaments stretch when under that kind of force, which inevitably leads to a weakened joint that will likely dislocate again and again.

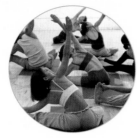
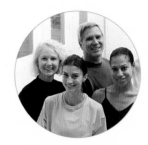
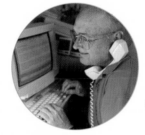
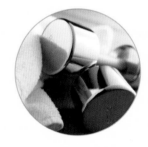
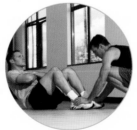
Tendons

Also known as sinews, tendons help the ligaments to stabilize and support the joints. These strong white cords of fibrous tissue serve to attach muscles to the bones of the joint. They work almost like springs, storing energy and adding support to a joint through the cycle of its normal movements (for example, the achilles tendon).

Muscles

Muscles provide the forces that move the bones within a joint. Even the simplest movement requires at least two muscles acting in equal and opposite ways: One contracts and pulls on its attached tendon, which in turn pulls on a bone to move it. At the same time, the opposing muscle relaxes to allow the movement to occur.

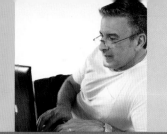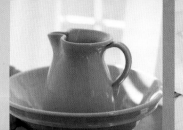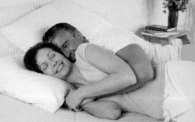

OSTEOARTHRITIS: cartilage gone bad

Osteoarthritis (OA) is by far the most common type of arthritis, affecting some three million Canadians, or about half of all Canadians with arthritis. Many people call it "old folks' arthritis," but it can happen to younger folks, too. Whatever your age, OA needs to be approached with an informed strategy so you can become an active participant in your own health care.

What Is OA?

"Osteo" is the Greek word for bone, and many people do think that OA is a bone disorder. But in actuality the condition mainly involves the cartilage that covers and cushions the ends of the bones within the joint.

> ➡ BONING UP: Osteoarthritis can occur in
>
> any joint in the body, but most commonly
>
> affects the hips, knees, lower back, neck and
>
> fingers. OA in the wrists, elbows and ankles
>
> can often be traced to an injury or to a job
>
> that subjects those joints to repeated stress.

Dysfunctional cartilage. In OA, the cartilage does not function as it was intended to and, for a variety of reasons, slowly breaks down. A number of possible causes—injury to the cartilage, genetic mutations, factors associated with aging—precipitate the breakdown. The result? The cartilage wears away—which is why osteoarthritis is sometimes referred to as "wear-and-tear" or "degenerative" arthritis. As the cartilage erodes, joints no longer move smoothly but instead feel—and sometimes sound—creaky.

Most OA sufferers have what is called primary OA, meaning the cause of their cartilage breakdown isn't known. In cases of secondary OA, cartilage damage can be traced to a specific cause such as a physical injury to the joint, misaligned bones or inflammation due to rheumatoid arthritis.

Unlike some other types of arthritis—rheumatoid arthritis, for instance—OA affects only the joints and not any other parts of the body. Not surprisingly, OA is most likely to develop in those joints that are subject to the greatest amount of stress: the body's weight-bearing joints, especially the knees and hips.

> ➡ BONING UP: If you have arthritis, there is a
>
> scientific name—crepitus—for the creaky feeling
>
> (and creaky noises) that you may notice when you
>
> move affected joints. Doctors feel —and listen—for
>
> signs of crepitus when diagnosing arthritis in patients.

Cartilage: The Inside Story

Water. Articular cartilage is mostly water—80 percent, in fact. Its high water content helps it to cushion the bones from trauma. Cartilage derives its water from the synovial fluid that bathes and lubricates the bones in a joint.

Collagen. This protein comes in the form of rod-shaped fibres that are the main building block for skin,

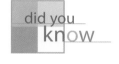

did you know

Osteoarthritis has been found in all mammals except those that spend most of their lives hanging upside down, like bats and sloths.

tendons, bones and other connective tissues. Collagen is a key ingredient in cartilage; strengthening it and helping it resist being pulled apart by pressure or other traumas.

Proteoglycans. Cartilage owes its high water content to proteoglycans—molecules that have the unique ability to soak up and hold fluid in the cartilage, allowing it to flow in and out as the pressure on a joint increases and decreases. Strands of proteoglycans team up with collagen to form a weblike, water-filled matrix that provides the cartilage with its spongelike resilience, its ability to absorb pressure and its surface slickness. OA begins with the breakdown of this matrix of proteoglycans and collagen.

Chondrocytes. Scattered throughout cartilage, these cells are responsible for synthesizing and repairing the cartilage "scaffolding"—namely, its collagen and proteoglycan molecules.

The road to osteoarthritis. As cartilage breaks down, it can no longer cushion bones or prevent them from rubbing against each other. In addition, bony swellings or spurs (known as osteophytes) may develop around the edge of bones in response to pressure on them. These changes lead to the symptoms that people with OA know all too well: pain, stiffness and restricted range of motion.

What Causes OA?

Again, the cause of primary osteoarthritis—what triggers joint cartilage erosion—is not yet known. The disease process apparently begins when destructive enzymes damage the network of collagen fibres that maintain the structure of cartilage. With its collagen "superstructure" damaged, cartilage swells with water, becoming softer and more vulnerable to stress and starting to wear away. Researchers have identified several risk factors that can significantly increase a person's odds of developing the disease:

Age. Age is the most powerful predictor of whether a person develops osteoarthritis. The condition is rare in young people, but becomes increasingly more common in older age groups. But don't misunderstand: though OA correlates with age, it isn't caused by it.

Instead, it now appears that factors associated with aging—and quite a few other factors as well—can make people susceptible to OA and cause their condition to worsen. Later chapters of this book will show you how to reduce all these risk factors.

Too many pounds. Wisdom isn't the only thing that increases with age. So does the waistline. Carrying around extra weight puts constant stress on the joints, eventually damaging the cartilage. This is particularly true for the weight-bearing joints: the knees and the hips.

If you're overweight, losing those extra kilos is one of the most effective of all osteoarthritis treatments available. A study that followed women of different weights over 36 years found that the heaviest women (those in the upper 20 percent by weight) were more than three times likelier than women in the bottom 20 percent to develop severe osteoarthritis of the knee. This was the first study showing that OA may be prevented.

Loose joints. When the bones of a joint aren't bound tightly to each other, they can bang together and damage their protective cartilage. Such "joint instability" is now recognized as a major cause of the pain and early-morning stiffness that may occur long before cartilage damage has begun. (Such symptoms are often felt by young, "double-jointed" women, whose flexibility makes them talented ballet dancers.) As a preventive measure, people with loose joints may be advised to avoid activities that could increase their risk of developing osteoarthritis prematurely.

On-the-job exertion. Certain jobs increase a person's risk for developing osteoarthritis. For example, OA of the knee is common among miners, dockworkers, people that must sit in a squat position over many years, as well as others who must constantly bend their knees or do heavy lifting. People in those professions are at risk of developing osteoarthritis of the knee.

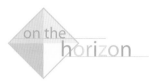

on the horizon

Researchers seeking the underlying cause of osteoarthritis have expanded their search beyond cartilage and into the underlying bone. Accumulating evidence suggests that changes in bone turnover—the counterbalancing process of bone breakdown and synthesis—may be involved in causing OA. British researcher Paul Dieppe has written that "Indeed, the cartilage may be the innocent bystander of a disease process that is centred more in bone than in cartilage.

Look to your genes. In 1990, after studying a family whose members developed osteoarthritis in many of their joints at a very early age, researchers reported on the first "osteoarthritis gene." They traced OA to a gene responsible for making the collagen in cartilage. A mutation in this gene causes the production of defective collagen, which probably weakens cartilage and causes it to break down prematurely.

Genes seem to influence osteoarthritis in particular joints as well. In 1944, researchers reported that OA involving the end joints of the fingers was an inherited trait. In this condition, small bony knobs known as Heberden's nodes (named after the eighteenth-century British physician who first described them) form on the top of the finger joints. Heberden's nodes are more common in women, particularly after menopause. Genes may also influence OA in other joints. In 1998, researchers studying 616 pairs of identical and fraternal female twins over age 40 concluded that genetic factors may be responsible for half of all cases of OA of the hip.

The estrogen factor. Women stand a much greater chance of developing osteoarthritis than men, especially as they get older. This gender difference is most extreme for OA of the knee in older people: Women over 65 are more than twice as likely to develop it as men the same age.

Couch potatoing. People tend to exercise less as they age—especially if they have arthritis. Unfortunately, inactivity itself increases your risk for osteoarthritis in several ways:

● Inactivity leads to weight gain, which puts extra strain on the joints.

● Tissues vital to joint movement—especially the muscles—can atrophy due to inactivity. Studies have shown that people with weak thigh muscles are more likely to develop OA of the knee.

● Inactivity can kill off chondrocytes, the cells that make and repair cartilage. Because cartilage has no blood vessels, chondrocytes must obtain nutrients from the synovial fluid. Walking or other weight-bearing activities contract and expand cartilage with each repetition, creating the pumping action of fluid vital for chondrocytes.

Taking a blow. The sports pages regularly report on athletes who've sustained serious injury to a joint—most often the knee. Unfortunately, an athlete or anyone else who suffers an injury to some part of a joint—cartilage, bone, ligament, or tendon—may eventually develop OA in that joint. With some injuries, such as a compound fracture of the ankle, osteoarthritis is almost a certainty. Pro athletes who incur frequent knee injuries will most likely develop OA of the knee after their playing days are over.

Joint by Joint: The Prime Targets of OA

Osteoarthritis can affect any of the body's joints, but it most often occurs in the hands, knees, hips or spine—or in joints that have been injured or stressed.

Hands. Osteoarthritis of the fingers is usually hereditary. Heberden's nodes, the small bony knobs that form on the ends of finger joints, occur most often in middle-aged and older women. The nodes are usually painless and tend to develop so slowly that a woman may not notice them until, for example, she has trouble slipping a ring over the joint.

Heberden's nodes are twice as likely to develop in women whose mothers also have them. Similar enlargements on the middle finger joints are known as Bouchard's nodes. Both Heberden's and Bouchard's nodes may first develop in one or a few fingers and later affect others. As Heberden himself noted, the problem with these nodes is mainly cosmetic.

caution

Early diagnosis and treatment is the best approach for any type of OA, but is especially important for OA of the knee. Treatment, including drugs, weight loss, exercise, hyaluronic acid injections and walking aids can all help prevent further joint damage. If left untreated, OA of the knee can become disabling, leaving joint replacement surgery as a patient's only recourse.

A more painful form of OA affecting the end joints of fingers is called nodal osteoarthritis. A single joint suddenly becomes painful, tender and swollen for three or four weeks—and then the problem subsides. Nodal OA is also hereditary and mainly affects women 45 and older, who are 10 times more likely to develop it than men in the same age group.

The joint at the base of the thumb also commonly develops osteoarthritis. By contrast, OA rarely affects the knuckles where the fingers attach to the hand.

Knees. The knees bear more weight than any other joint in the body—which makes them very susceptible to OA. When that happens, the knees may become swollen and feel stiff when you try to move them. You may notice you have trouble walking to the mailbox, climbing stairs and getting in and out of the car. According to studies, strengthening the muscles surrounding the knee can often dramatically improve the symptoms of osteoarthritis of the knee.

Hips. Like the knees, the weight-bearing hips are susceptible to OA. People with osteoarthritis of the hip may have trouble bending and the pain and stiffness

DO YOU HAVE OSTEOARTHRITIS? MONITOR YOUR SYMPTOMS

■ One or more joints has a deep and aching pain that is steady or intermittent

■ Pain is worsened by exercise or other activities and eased by rest

■ Joint pain develops that won't go away, even after resting the joint for several days

■ One or more joints feels stiff for 30 minutes or less after you get out of bed

■ One or more joints swells or feels tender

■ Affected joint has grinding feeling or makes a grinding sound

■ When you start moving after sitting during the day—after driving a fairly long distance or seeing a movie, for example—you feel stiff for the next 20 or 30 minutes

may cause them to limp when they walk. The pain may not only be felt in the hip but may also radiate to other parts of the body, especially the groin or down the inside of the thigh. As we've already said, some cases of osteoarthritis of the hip seem to be hereditary. Also, people who are bowlegged or who have other congenital abnormalities that cause the bones of the hip to be misaligned are at increased risk for hip osteoarthritis.

Losing weight can help—but is not as helpful for relieving hip osteoarthritis as it is for the knee. Drugs and exercise can also help relieve pain and improve movement. Hip-replacement surgery is very effective when other treatments fall short of relieving the pain or disability.

Spine. Osteoarthritis of the spine mainly causes stiffness and pain in the neck or in the lower back. Measures that can help relieve the symptoms include exercises that strengthen the muscles of the back and abdomen; heat treatments; and the use of support pillows when sitting. In some people, bone spurs growing from the edges of the vertebrae may squeeze the spinal nerves, causing pain, weakness or numbness in the arms or legs. When this happens, surgery may be necessary to relieve the pressure on the nerves.

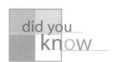

did you know

How Does OA Progress?

The breakdown of cartilage that leads to OA does not occur overnight, even though that first sharp pain in your knee might make it seem to come on all of a sudden. No, this erosion almost always happens slowly, over many months

Experts now believe that morning stiffness (also known as gelling) results from the accumulation of synovial fluid inside the joint while the person with arthritis is asleep. Once the person wakes up and starts moving, the excess fluid is pumped out and the stiffness subsides.

or years, as the once-smooth cartilage becomes thinner, develops a roughened surface and loses its cushioning ability.

Sometimes, the pain and stiffness that accompany the disintegrating cartilage appears so gradually that people ignore it or chalk it up to "getting older." And for many lucky people, this is as far as their osteoarthritis ever progresses: In those cases it remains a only mild problem; causing symptoms they're barely aware of.

When cartilage continues to erode, however, the increasingly bothersome symptoms send many people to the doctor's office. After exercise, knees and other joints may ache or feel stiff for a brief time. You may also feel stiff after you've been sitting for awhile—for example, when climbing out of the car after a long ride or getting up after watching a movie.

Bone meets bone. Eventually, cartilage wears away to the point that, in some areas, the bones rub up against one another. People may feel their knees lock briefly as they climb the stairs, or they might experience a grinding sensation—or even hear a grinding sound—when they bend affected knees or hips. People may also find themselves avoiding once-routine activities because of the pain—the daily walk to the newsstand, for example, or working in the garden on weekends. If the affected joint is a hip or knee, people may begin to limp as they try to minimize the pain.

Furthermore, small chunks of fragmented cartilage floating in the synovial fluid may begin to irritate the synovial membrane and add to the discomfort. In response, the membrane becomes inflamed and produces excess fluid, which makes the joint swell. In addition to pain, a person may now notice that the joint's range of motion is becoming restricted.

Bone spurs and other painful growths. OA becomes more severe as changes extend beyond cartilage to the underlying bones, which may sprout small growths (known as bone spurs or osteophytes) around their outer edges. Bone spurs increase the joint's surface area and may be the bones' defensive reaction to the extra pressure created when their protective covering has worn away.

Unfortunately, bone spurs often make things worse: Spurs on the spine, for example, may cause severe pain by pinching the nerves connecting the spinal cord to the muscles; sharp spurs around the rim of the knee joint may worsen the pain and tenderness. By this time, people may find that arthritis pain is keeping them awake at night.

When the cartilage is completely eroded, the sensitive bones rub against each other within the joint. At this point, the pain can be excruciating and nearly unrelenting even after the slightest movement. When such severe osteoarthritis affects weight-bearing joints—like the knees or the hips—it can be crippling, especially if:

● Uneven cartilage loss has created uneven joint surfaces, causing bones to become misaligned, leading to instability in the joint itself.

● Extensive bone-spur formation limits the affected joint's mobility.

● The muscles and tendons that support the joint have shortened and weakened due to disuse, leading to muscle spasms and even more disability. Today's joint-replacement operations can be a godsend for people with such severe osteoarthritis.

How is OA diagnosed

Relief for your pain starts with an accurate diagnosis as this gets you off on the right track for treatment. For doctors familiar with OA, telling whether you have the disease usually isn't difficult. A comprehensive diagnosis is based on a doctor taking your clinical history, doing a physical exam and running some tests.

Clinical history. The doctor will ask you a series of questions to get information about your symptoms—when they started, where they occur, what they feel like, whether they've changed over time and how they're affecting your life. The doctor will also ask about other diseases you may have (which could be the cause of your symptoms) and drugs you may be taking (which may interfere with some anti–arthritis drugs).

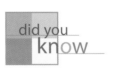

did you know

Osteoarthritis pain tends to worsen toward the end of the day. In many other types or arthritis, the pain remains constant during the day or is worse in the morning.

Doctors have found that answers to three questions in particular provide a good gauge of whether a patient has arthritis (or some other musculoskeletal disease) and how severely disabled he or she is:

● Do you have any pain or stiffness in your muscles, joints or back?

● Can you dress yourself completely without difficulty?

● Can you walk up and down stairs without difficulty?

The doctor then follows up any positive answers with more specific questions. The discussion should also cover:

Pain: The location of the pain, its severity, character, and timing.

Stiffness: No other condition causes the same type of joint stiffness as osteoarthritis.

Swelling: Eighty-five to 90 percent of people with osteoarthritis don't experience swelling. However, swelling can indicate the degree of joint damage or suggest that there's another problem.

Severity: The degree of pain suggests joint damage and how much treatment you may need.

Causes: Knowing if you suffered an injury before the pain started is a valuable clue that you are suffering from secondary OA. If no injury occurred, chances increase that you have primary osteoarthritis.

The physical exam

Following a routine exam to assess your overall health (taking your blood pressure, listening to your heart and so on), the doctor will focus on the joints that are bothering you—feeling and pressing on them for signs of swelling or tenderness and watching how they work when you walk or bend. The doctor will also assess other joints, which could be affected by arthritis even though you don't know it yet.

---

caution

If your doctor skimps on either the conversation or the physical exam and tries to diagnose or rule out osteoarthritis on X-rays alone, find yourself another doctor.

Taking your medical history as part of the initial visit is a crucial part of the diagnostic process, since it can help your doctor determine what type of arthritis you have and choose the right laboratory tests to confirm the diagnosis. You can do your doctor and yourself a big favour by arriving well prepared. Try to bring:

■ Your medical records, including copies of recent X-rays and blood tests

■ A list of other medical problems that you have

■ A list of all the drugs you take—prescription and over-the-counter as well as herbs or other dietary supplements

■ A written "narrative" in which you describe your problem as fully as you can, including: how long ago the joint pain began, whether the symptoms came on suddenly or slowly, which joints were initially affected, what triggered the symptoms (e.g., exercise, climbing stairs, etc.) and the activities most strongly impacted by your joint pain.

During the joint examination, the doctor will ask you to move joints (known as active motion) and will also move them himself (passive motion). In true joint disease, movement is limited and causes pain with both active and passive motion. If the doctor can move a joint further than you can (flex your knee in a wider arc, for example), then you probably don't have a problem with your joint but instead with the tendons or muscles surrounding it.

Different joints are examined in different ways:

Hands. The doctor checks for bony enlargements on the end joints of fingers or on the middle joints. These nodes are clear signs of osteoarthritis.

Hips. Limited range of motion is the key indicator. With the patient lying on his back with knees bent, the doctor places one hand on the knee and the other on the heel and then rotates the foot outward and inward. Restricted inward rotation is typically an early sign of hip osteoarthritis.

Knees. In addition to checking for abnormalities in joint movement, the doctor looks for areas of swelling around the knee joint.

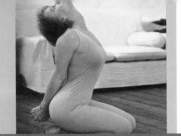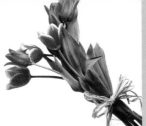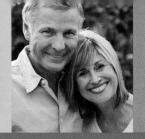

RHEUMATOID ARTHRITIS:
fire in the joints

Rheumatoid arthritis (RA) is the most common type of inflammatory arthritis, and usually affects many joints in the body. RA is much less common than osteoarthritis, affecting only about one percent of Canadians (some 300,000 people), with women accounting for three of every four people with the disease. RA can begin at any age, but most commonly develops in young and middle-aged adults.

What Is RA?

RA is a systemic disease. What this means is that RA can affect not only the joints but also the blood vessels, heart, skin, muscles and other parts of the body. Most people with RA must contend with daily pain and stiffness, which may wax and wane. They often speak of having good days and bad days, weeks or months and of enduring periods of depression, anxiety and helplessness. In these cases, a self-empowerment approach can play a central role in helping people with RA gain control over their disease and their lives.

Do you really have it? RA and osteoarthritis are often mistaken for each other—which can cause serious problems, since the two types of arthritis are

RA VERSUS OA: COMPARISONS & CONTRASTS

Age of occurrence. Rheumatoid arthritis (RA) usually develops between the ages of 20 and 50, but can occur at any age. Osteoarthritis (OA) is a disease of middle and old age and rarely occurs before age 45.

Pattern of disease. RA often strikes symmetrically, meaning it affects both wrists, the knuckles on both hands, etc. OA rarely affects both joints (e.g., both wrists) at once.

Speed of onset. About 20 percent of RA cases develop suddenly, within weeks or months. OA develops slowly, with cartilage breakdown usually occurring over several years.

Extent of illness. In addition to causing joint damage, RA can cause fatigue, fever, anemia and weight loss and damage the heart and other organs. OA is limited to the joints.

Joints affected. RA usually affects many joints, including the wrists (which are affected in almost all RA cases), knuckles, elbows, shoulders, ankles, feet and neck (but usually spares the rest of the spine). OA most commonly affects the knees, hips, feet, hands and spine; sometimes affects the knuckles and wrists; and rarely affects the elbows and shoulders.

Hand involvement. RA affects many of the hand joints, but usually not the knuckles closest to the fingernails. OA affects the knuckles closest to the fingernails more often than other joints of the hand.

Morning stiffness. People with RA have prolonged morning stiffness, usually lasting for at least 30 minutes after they get up. With OA, morning stiffness lasts less than 30 minutes.

treated quite differently. Although symptoms may be similar, RA and OA are very different diseases.

Osteoarthritis can affect any joint that has cartilage—freely movable joints such as the knee or slightly movable joints like the vertebrae. By contrast, RA focuses on the body's freely movable joints and on one area in particular: the synovial membrane, which is the inner lining of the capsule surrounding freely movable joints. Once this joint becomes inflamed, the characteristic symptoms of rheumatoid arthritis—heat, swelling, stiffness and pain—begin to appear.

> ➡ BONING UP: If you have arthritis, you may
>
> swear that your stiffness and pain get worse when
>
> the weather changes. And they probably do. Studies
>
> using climate chambers have found that people with
>
> arthritis really do experience increased stiffness and
>
> pain when the barometric pressure drops quickly or
>
> when the humidity suddenly rises.

While osteoarthritis confines its damage to the joints, RA is a systemic disease that can damage not only the joints but also other parts of the body such as blood vessels, the eyes and the heart. This tissue damage is caused by chronic inflammation—the hallmark of RA. Although inflammation can also occur in osteoarthritis, it is confined to the affected joints.

What Causes RA?

The causes of RA's key feature—chronic inflammation—are not known. However, scientists do know that a glitch in the immune system is involved. Like psoriasis, lupus, multiple sclerosis and type I diabetes, RA is an autoimmune disease, meaning that the body's immune system mistakenly attacks healthy tissue as if it were a foreign invader.

RA's target. This autoimmune attack is directed against the joint's synovial membrane. It inflames the joint and causes pain, warmth, stiffness and swelling—symptoms common to many types of arthritis. What makes RA different from other forms of inflammatory arthritis is the potential for the inflamed synovial membrane to severely damage the joints.

If that's not enough, RA's inflammation may spread beyond the joints to affect other parts of the body. Fortunately, new disease-modifying drugs can block RA's spread by inactivating the immune system components that attack the body's own tissues.

Researchers have identified risk factors that make some people more likely to develop RA than others. Chief among these risk factors is a person's genetic makeup.

The role of heredity

It seems that many people who develop RA inherited their susceptibility to the disease. Several different genes probably determine whether someone will have a tendency to develop RA and how severe his or her disease will be. As you might expect, these tend to be genes that control the immune system.

For example, some 65 percent of people with RA have a genetic marker—a protein called HLA-DR4—on the surface of their white blood cells. White cells play major roles in the body's effort to fight infections, so this protein may somehow trick white cells into attacking the body's own tissues.

A missing link. Patients who have this genetic marker usually have more severe RA than those patients without it. However, fully one in four people who have the marker never develop RA, which shows that having "RA genes" isn't sufficient to bring on the condition. Instead, researchers believe something must be present to trigger RA in susceptible people.

The search for a trigger. For a century now, researchers have searched for a link between the onset of RA and literally dozens of infectious agents. It used to be that bacteria were the prime suspects: Since they

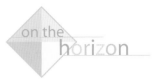

on the horizon

A treatment that may actually cure rheumatoid arthritis was reported back in late 2000 at the annual scientific meeting of the American College of Rheumatology. Developed by researchers at University College in London, the treatment involves depleting the blood of B-lymphocytes; these immune cells form antibodies that cause much of the joint destruction that occurs in RA. Even now, research is still ongoing, but B lymphocyte depletion still looks good as a treatment option.

were implicated in causing some types of arthritis (Reiter's syndrome, for instance), it made sense that bacteria could be involved in RA as well.

In 1912, an American rheumatologist proposed that RA occurred when bacterial toxins from localized infections in the tonsils, gums, teeth, or gallbladder were carried to the joints via the bloodstream. This focal infection theory failed to hold water, but for the next 30 years unfortunate RA patients had their tonsils removed or all their teeth pulled in a vain effort to halt the progress of the disease.

To see if RA was contagious, researchers in 1950 took fluid from the joints of people with RA and injected it into the joints of healthy volunteers. None of the volunteers developed RA—conclusive evidence that RA does not involve a persistent infection of the joints.

In recent years, viruses have received the most attention as possible culprits in triggering RA. One prime suspect for more than a decade has been the Epstein-Barr virus, which causes mononucleosis. Studies show that susceptible people—those with any one of three genes associated with RA—tend to have an abnormal immune response to Epstein-Barr infections, which may trigger RA.

Many arthritis experts remain convinced that infections can initiate RA. So far, the strenuous efforts to link a bacterium, virus, or some other infectious agent to the condition have all failed. But even if some microbe is eventually implicated in causing RA, one thing seems certain: You can't catch RA from someone else.

➡ BONING UP: Rheumatoid arthritis can affect
any of the body's freely movable joints, but most
commonly involves the hands, wrists, shoulders,
elbows, knees, ankles and feet.

The estrogen factor

Women are much more susceptible to autoimmune diseases than men—and RA is no exception: Three of every four people who develop RA are women, and researchers suspect that estrogen is the culprit. Combined with certain "susceptibility genes," estrogen seems to tip the balance toward developing RA: For example, a woman who inherits the genes will very likely develop the disease, while a brother with the same genes will remain healthy. When a woman has a genetic tendency to develop RA, estrogen may super-sensitize her immune system so that—in response to some infection—immune cells launch an attack on her tissues and the invading microbes.

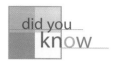

Recent studies suggest that fewer people are developing rheumatoid arthritis than in previous years, but no one knows the reason why.

How Does RA Progress?

In about 80 percent of cases, RA begins slowly, affecting just a few joints at first, typically those in the fingers, wrists or toes. Eventually, the disease almost always ends up affecting 20 joints or more, including the shoulders, ankles, hips, knees and other joints. But not all cases develop gradually: RA sometimes appears seemingly overnight, involving many of the body's joints in just a matter of days.

If inflammation persists, the synovial membrane's cells may start to grow uncontrollably, forming extra tissue called pannus and thickening the normally thin membrane. The joint becomes swollen and feels puffy to the touch.

A slow cascade of pain. As RA progresses, the growing synovial membrane spreads and eventually covers the top of the joint cartilage. Invading cells from the thickened, inflamed synovial membrane release destructive enzymes that erode the cartilage and underlying bone of the joint and eventually weaken the muscles, tendons and ligaments that surround it.

In RA's later stages, joints can become so severely damaged that they no longer function properly. The inflammation may totally erode the cartilage and deform a joint by causing bones to fuse together. Fortunately, today's disease-modifying anti-rheumatic drugs can prevent crippling and disability in many cases—if treatment begins early enough.

How Is RA Diagnosed?

RA can be notoriously difficult to diagnose, especially in its early stages. Its symptoms usually don't appear all at once, but typically reveal themselves slowly over a

THE FOUR DEGREES OF RA

No two cases of RA proceed in exactly the same way. In fact, experts stress that RA's course in any patient is quite unpredictable. But they have identified four basic ways that the disease progresses—or, in some cases, doesn't.

1. In a few people—perhaps around 10 percent who develop it—RA is a temporary problem: These people experience a spontaneous and lasting remission that can't be attributed to any treatment they might be undergoing. When they happen, these spontaneous remissions usually occur within the first two years that people have RA. Another 10 percent of RA patients experience remissions, but the disease recurs later.

2. In the second type of RA, patients experience periodic flare-ups—weeks or months of painful, stiff and swollen joints—that alternate with intervals of normal health. Their treatment will depend on whether their joints are damaged during the flare-ups and how well their joints function between flare-ups.

3. In the third type of RA, known as remitting-progressive, patients experience periodic flare-ups without returning to normal health between the attacks. Instead, during the periods between attacks, they have lingering joint inflammation that becomes increasingly more severe with each attack. If it isn't treated properly, remitting-progressive RA can eventually lead to significant joint damage.

4. The fourth type is called progressive RA, which is self-explanatory: The inflammation becomes more severe over time and causes gradually increasing pain, swelling, and—if severe inflammation lasts long enough—joint damage and disability.

period of months or years. Stiff, painful joints are usually among the first symptoms of RA, but they also occur in many other joint diseases. For this reason, diagnosing RA often requires ruling out other possible causes of the symptoms.

Medical history

As with OA, the first step is for a doctor to take your medical history (see page 17). The answers to certain questions, like "Which joints are giving you trouble?" or "Do the joints feel stiff in the morning and, if so, how long does the stiffness last?" can help a doctor narrow the list of possible joint problems.

Physical exam

The doctor will focus on the affected joints, looking for the telltale signs of RA: joints with a limited range of motion and that are tender, reddened, swollen or warm. As noted earlier, problems in symmetrical joints—both elbows, for example—increase the odds that RA is present.

Lab test

Only one laboratory test is useful for confirming a diagnosis of RA: the rheumatoid factor test. Rheumatoid factor is an antibody produced by the synovial membranes of joints affected by RA, and can be found in the blood of 80 to 90 percent of people with the condition. (Unfortunately, rheumatoid factor is often absent in the early stages of RA—when the test's help in diagnosing the disease is most needed.) In general, patients who test positive for rheumatoid factor tend to have more severe RA than those who test negative, and people with high levels of rheumatoid factor are more acutely affected than those with low amounts.

It's in the blood. Another test, the erythrocyte sedimentation rate, or "sed rate," is a broad indicator of inflammation in the body, including RA. Inflammation tends to make red blood cells sticky, so they form

RHEUMATIC RUNDOWN

Painful, swollen joints occur in a large number of joint ailments. Here is a rundown of rheumatic diseases with similar symptoms:

- Rheumatoid arthritis
- Ankylosing spondylitis
- Systemic lupus erythematosus
- Arthritis associated with psoriasis
- Reiter's syndrome
- Gout
- Pseudogout
- Bursitis

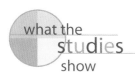

what the studies show

A large-scale study published in 1994 found that an average of nine months elapsed between the time RA patients first noticed symptoms and when they were finally diagnosed with RA.

clumps that will settle ("sediment out") in a test tube. The greater the inflammation, the larger the red-cell clumps and the faster they'll fall to the bottom of the tube. This makes the sed rate useful for monitoring whether a treatment for RA is reducing inflammation. But because infections, malignancies and other problems can provoke inflammation, the sed rate is not useful for initially diagnosing the condition.

An inside job. A useful but more invasive way to confirm that a person has some form of inflammatory arthritis is to evaluate synovial fluid removed from an affected joint by use of a needle. The fluid is examined for neutrophils, which are the white blood cells that gather at sites of inflammation.

X-rays

These are not the best way to diagnose RA. They often appear totally normal early in the course of the disease, even when symptoms are severe. In fact, X-rays usually don't provide evidence of RA until significant and irreversible joint damage has occurred. At that point, X-rays reveal that inflammation has destroyed cartilage and eroded the underlying bone.

What Now?

A diagnosis of RA can be sobering: The disease can cause significant joint damage and disability. It can disrupt people's lives, affecting their relationships and draining their financial resources as it affects their work situations. But you can blunt RA's impact if you approach the disease in the right way.

Don't panic. The great majority of people who are diagnosed with RA have relatively mild symptoms that can be controlled with proper treatment. Furthermore, breakthrough treatments for RA have been introduced in just the past few years, and the pace of research indicates that and even better treatments are on the horizon.

Tell your friends and family. Even people with mild cases of RA can expect to experience periodic flares—sudden worsening of the inflammation that can temporarily disable a person with pain and fatigue. If family and friends are aware of this and other RA-related complications, they'll be more understanding and more willing to pitch in to help when you're not feeling up to par.

Choose the right doctor. If you've been diagnosed with RA, you owe it to yourself and your family to be treated by a rheumatologist, a physician who specializes in treating rheumatoid and other types of arthritis. More than most other diseases, RA demands close monitoring and fine-tuning of treatment to prevent permanent joint damage. You need a doctor who is experienced in treating RA and who is familiar with the latest treatments.

SURVIVING FLARE-UPS

What is a flare-up? For people diagnosed with any type of arthritis, the word "flare" becomes an important part of their vocabulary. Things may be going along smoothly—so smoothly you've almost forgotten you have arthritis—and then, suddenly, a flare.

■ Arthritis flares are times when things go bad: inflammation, pain and stiffness resurface with a vengeance. Flares can be set off by many different things—overdoing it at the gym, lack of sleep or even emotional stress.

■ Flares can severely challenge the patience—sometimes even the sanity—of people with arthritis. Successfully taking charge of arthritis means riding out a flare so that it causes the least amount of aggravation and despair.

Minimizing pain. The key is learning how to adjust to a flare without giving in to it. When a flare comes on, you'll want to give yourself more rest and protect the inflamed joints from further exertion. On the other hand, overprotecting a joint can be counterproductive, since long periods of inactivity can cause the muscles and tendons around a joint to weaken. You may also want to consult with your doctor about adjusting your medication in response to a flare.

Unfortunately, flares are an unavoidable part of arthritis. But knowing you can manage these periodic crises means you don't have to live in dread of them.

Until the late 1980s, doctors believed that early RA could be managed exclusively with NSAIDs and that disease-modifying anti-rheumatic drugs (DMARDs) weren't needed until joint damage showed up on X-rays. They later realized that permanent joint damage can occur even in the first months of RA—despite the use of NSAIDs and long before damage can be seen on X-rays. Now, experts agree that use of DMARDs should begin almost as soon as RA is diagnosed

It is also important to choose a doctor you feel comfortable with, since the two of you will be working closely to develop an effective treatment plan.

Assemble a health-care team. In general, people with RA do best under the care of several health-care professionals. In addition to your physician, you may benefit from working with a physiotherapist (who can help you set up an exercise program) and a psychologist or mental-health professional (who can steer you through the periods of depression and helplessness that RA patients may experience from time to time).

In RA, patient and doctor work together to achieve several goals:

● To alleviate pain, stiffness, swelling, fatigue and other symptoms

● To reduce the inflammation

● To slow down or halt the joint damage

● To limit RA's interference with a patient's life

Set realistic goals. This is important for people with any type of arthritis—but especially RA, a disease that can pose significant physical and emotional challenges.

caution

Today, someone diagnosed with RA can expect to receive early and aggressive treatment with powerful drugs that can have serious side effects: all the more reason, experts say, to avoid a rush to diagnostic judgment. When the presence of RA is unclear, the best of all diagnostic tests is the test of time. It may take a few weeks or months of repeated assessment, but a true case of RA will eventually reveal itself.

FILTERING OUT RA

In March 2000 Health Canada approved the Prosorba column, the first non-drug alternative for adults with moderate to severe RA who cannot tolerate disease-modifying anti-rheumatic drugs (DMARDs). During a two-hour process, the patient's blood is removed and passed through a machine that separates the plasma (liquid part of the blood) from the blood cells. The plasma is then passed through the Prosorba column, a device about the size of a coffee mug. The filtered plasma is then recombined with its blood cells, and the blood is reinfused into the patient.

The Prosorba treatment (once a week for 12 weeks) can cause dramatic improvement in RA patients. Although researchers don't fully understand the column's mechanism of action, they believe it filters out proteins involved in the immune system's attack on the joints.

Setting and meeting realistic goals is vital to coping with the condition.

Make use of resources. People with RA can benefit greatly from a wide variety of resources, including the programs and self-help courses sponsored by their local Arthritis Society chapter, as well as support groups and health information offered on the Internet.

Drugs can put out the fire

Virtually all people diagnosed with RA must rely on drugs to control their disease. The arsenal of drugs falls generally into two classes: NSAIDs (nonsteroidal anti-inflammatory drugs) and DMARDs (disease-modifying anti-rheumatic drugs). Successful treatment of RA usually requires the person with RA to take both types. For more information on the drugs available to you, see The Medical Arsenal (p. 45).

Surgery: A new lease on mobility

When RA's joint damage is severe, there are several types of surgical repair that can be performed. For more about surgical RA treatment, see Surgery: A New Lease on Mobility (p. 48).

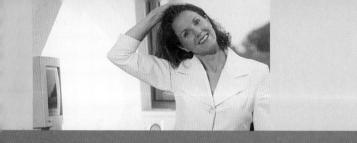
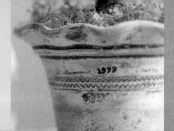
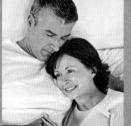

FIBROMYALGIA:
it's not just in your mind

If you literally ache all over, you may have fibromyalgia (FM)—one of the most vexing of all medical problems. One recent textbook described FM as a "chronic, poorly understood and disabling condition." It is all of that and perhaps more.

FM is relatively common, affecting about 900,000 Canadians, or just under three percent of the general population. The overwhelming majority of FM patients are women (by a 4-to-1 ratio) and the ailment typically strikes when a person is over 50. Fibromyalgia is a significant health problem, accounting for one of every six visits that people make to rheumatologists.

What Is FM?

FM's main features are severe and widespread muscle pain that is most pronounced in the neck and shoulders, extreme fatigue and—in most cases—poor sleep. Fibromyalgia can feel like a joint disease, but the pain actually occurs in nearby muscles, ligaments and tendons.

FM's pain and other symptoms may persist for years—even for life—but the intensity can vary from day to day. Both inactivity and unaccustomed physical activity can make symptoms worse, as can insomnia, humid weather and emotional stress.

In addition to widespread persistent pain, fatigue and poor sleep, people with FM typically report many other problems including:

● Irritable bowel syndrome (present in up to 50 percent of cases)

● Tension headaches

● Problems concentrating or remembering

● A sense of swollen hands, though examination shows the hands to be normal

● Palpitations

● Depression

What Causes FM?

One of the most frustrating aspects of FM—for patients, their families and their doctors—is the absence of any definite cause or causes. FM may well be the result of a complex interaction among many different physiological and psychological factors. For now, experts have proposed a number of theories for what causes FM, including:

Heredity

Research shows that FM patients are more likely than other people to have a family history of pain, depression or alcoholism. Not surprisingly, FM is more common among relatives of FM patients than among relatives of nonaffected people.

Until about 20 years ago FM was known as fibrositis, a condition of inflamed ("-itis") muscles, tendons, and other fibrous tissues. In 1979, Canadian physicians showed that fibrositis patients also suffered from extreme fatigue and, in almost all cases, problems with sleep. Studies also found that achy joints of fibrositis patients were not actually inflamed. So in 1981 Dr. Muhammad B. Yunus, professor of medicine at the University of Illinois College of Medicine at Peoria, specifically used the 1976 term "fibromyalgia," which roughly means achy muscles and other soft tissues. The World Health Organization recognized FM as a medical disorder in its Copenhagen Declaration of New Year's Day 1993.

Stress

Most researchers agree that stress is a key factor in FM. Studies show that FM patients report high levels of stress in their lives—more, for example, than in RA patients or in other non-FM sufferers.

A recent study involving FM patients found that the greater their psychological distress, the more sensitive they are to pain and the more physical complaints they have. What's not clear is whether stress causes FM or is the consequence of living with a severe and sometimes disabling condition.

A real problem. Even if stress causes FM, the disorder clearly isn't "all in the mind," as some sceptics contend, but is a genuine medical problem. Mind-body research over the past decade shows that emotional stress can cause major changes in the body and adversely affect the nervous system, immune system and hormone levels.

High levels of substance P

Responsible for alerting the nervous system to a painful injury of the tissues, elevated levels of the chemical known as "substance P" are found in the cerebrospinal fluid of FM patients. In some people with FM, levels of substance P consistently measure two to three times above normal; in others, substance P levels gradually increase as symptoms become more severe. Increased substance P levels, perhaps induced by stress, may help explain the recent finding that FM patients have lower pain thresholds than people who don't have the condition.

Injury, accident or trauma

Some people can trace the onset of their FM to relatively minor accidents such as fender-bender collisions. But most experts doubt that minor trauma can produce the long-lasting effects on muscles and other soft tissue throughout the body that characterizes FM.

How Is FM Diagnosed?

A striking feature of FM is that standard diagnostic tests—blood chemistries or X-rays, for example—appear perfectly normal. As a result, a diagnosis of FM must be made by clinical examination. In 1990, after comparing FM patients with control patients, the American College of Rheumatology set out specific criteria for physicians to use in diagnosing FM. These criteria are used by Canadian doctors when making an FM diagnosis. To be diagnosed with FM, patients must have:

- Widespread muscle pain that has been present for at least three months
- Pain in at least 11 of 18 "tender points" when a doctor pushes on those spots

➡ BONING UP: Next to osteoarthritis, FM is the second most commonly diagnosed musculosketel disorder.

What Now?

If you're like many people, you may actually be relieved to receive a diagnosis of FM: Some people spend years seeking an explanation for their symptoms, with numerous doctors telling them that the problem is all in their head.

Since there is no known cause for FM, treatment is aimed at easing its symptoms, which is not an easy task. For example, drugs that work well at relieving pain associated with many types of arthritic problems—

TAKING CHARGE OF FIBROMYALGIA

Sometimes it's easier to have a clear-cut medical problem than one like FM, with its largely subjective symptoms of pain and fatigue. People with FM must often contend with sceptical doctors and family members who doubt whether their complaints are real.

Hands-on benefits. For this and other reasons—including a lack of truly effective treatments—FM can be an especially difficult illness to cope with, but also one that can be greatly helped by the take-charge approach espoused in this book. Studies consistently show that by gaining self-empowerment—believing in your ability to control your disease and overcome symptoms—FM patients can improve their mood, decrease pain and better tolerate the pain they still have.

ibuprofen and other NSAIDs—are notably ineffective against the pain of fibromyalgia. The difficulty involved in finding effective treatments often only adds to the frustration that many FM patients experience. Applying topical treatments (p. 46) seems to work well for some people with FM, as does acupuncture (p. 47).

Accentuate the positive. The upside for people with FM is that it doesn't involve damage to the joints. Even though you may hurt all over and feel exhausted, you won't be crippled by FM. On the other hand, FM tends to linger—sometimes for life—although the severity of the pain and fatigue may ebb and flow over the years. One of the keys to coping with FM is overcoming the sleep disturbances that contribute to FM's sometimes disabling fatigue.

Exercise. Although no single treatment has proven universally effective against FM, physicians who have cared for many FM patients seem to agree that aerobic exercise should be a part of any treatment program. For one thing, aerobic exercise improves sleep—almost always poor among FM patients—and better sleep helps relieve FM's extreme fatigue. In addition, studies show that aerobic exercise helps to ease muscle pain and tenderness in FM patients.

Many fibromyalgia patients find that a combination of different treatments is the best route to relief for their symptoms. Other possible treatments for FM include:

The chemical cure. Low does of antidepressants, as well as NSAIDs and topical treatments are the established medicines for treating FM. To read up on these aids, see The Medical Arsenal (p. 45).

caution

FM patients embarking on an exercise regimen should start out slowly, especially if they've been inactive, since unaccustomed exertion can cause severe pain. You should also avoid high-impact exercises—jogging or tennis, for example—and opt for road biking, walking or swimming instead.

Routine maintenance. Other things you can do to regulate your condition are:

● Eat several small meals during the day to maintain a steady supply of protein and carbohydrate for proper muscle function.

● Take hot baths or showers—especially in the morning—to soothe soreness, increase circulation and relieve stiffness.

● Find a massage therapist familiar with fibromyalgia. A technique called trigger-point therapy can be extremely helpful in reducing pain.

● Cut back on caffeine, alcohol and sugar, all of which often cause fatigue.

● Get at least eight hours of sleep a night.

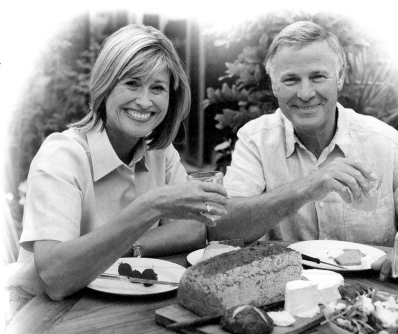

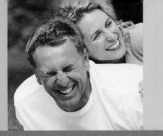

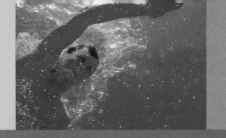

ANKYLOSING SPONDYLITIS:
back pain with a twist

Anywhere from 150,000 to 300,000 Canadians (up to one in 100) are believed to suffer from Ankylosing Spondylitis (AS), a chronic inflammation of the spine. It is three times more common in men than in women, but recent research suggests that the ratio may be much more equal: women often have much milder cases that usually escape detection.

AS is mainly a disease of young people, often beginning before age 20 and rarely affecting people over 40. Once thought to be part of rheumatoid arthritis, we now know that it is related but separate.

What Is AS?

AS is a type of chronic arthritis that mainly affects the spine. (*Ankylosing* means stiff, *spondyl* refers to the spine and *itis* means inflammation.) In AS, the inflammation occurs in joints and in areas where tendons and ligaments attach to bones. In severe cases, inflammation of the spine can actually cause the spinal vertebrae to fuse.

Older people who walk hunched over, looking down at the ground are usually in the late stages of AS. The good news is that today's treatment approaches can almost always prevent AS from becoming a disabling or crippling condition.

What Causes AS?

As with many types of arthritis, the cause of AS is not known. But genes have a strong influence, since AS occurs primarily in people who have a genetic marker, or protein, called HLA-B27 on the surface of their white blood cells. Someone who carries the HLA-B27 gene has a one to two percent risk of developing AS—but the risk can rise to 20 percent if a first-degree relative (parent or sibling) has the disease.

How Does AS Progress?

AS typically begins gradually, almost insidiously. The first symptoms are usually aches and pains in the lower back caused by inflammation of the sacroiliac joints, located in the lower back on both sides of the spine, just above the buttocks (lower back pain that begins gradually and persists for months is often a tip-off for the disease). The backache can be quite severe, interfering with sleep and causing a person to roll sideways to avoid bending the back when getting out of bed.

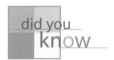

Ankylosing spondylitis can be traced to antiquity. In 1912, archaeologists unearthed an Egyptian mummy from about 3,000 BCE, which showed signs of severe AS. The mummy's spine was described as "a rigid block of stone" extending from its base to the neck.

➡ BONING UP: One way to distinguish between a ruptured disk and early ankylosing spondylitis is that while disk pain is improved with rest, the pain of AS usually gets worse with rest and better with movement.

Ascending pain. As it progresses, AS and its inflammation may move to the upper back or spread to other joints, especially the neck, hips and shoulders. The spine becomes stiff due to pain and muscle spasms. In the final stages of AS, chronic inflammation can cause bony bridges to form between the vertebrae, resulting in the spine fusing permanently into a bent and inflexible position.

AS is a systemic disease, so it sometimes affects areas of the body beyond the joints. People with AS may experience fatigue, weight loss, poor appetite and—in about 25 percent of patients—an inflammatory eye condition known as iritis, which causes redness and tearing. People with severe and long-standing AS may experience damage to heart tissue that requires the implantation of a pacemaker.

How Is AS Diagnosed?

Ankylosing spondylitis can be a challenging disease to diagnose, especially in its early stages. In general, the medical history alone can offer a doctor several clues that, when pieced together, point to a diagnosis of AS:

● The patient is a male between 16 and 35

● Back pain and stiffness developed gradually

● Symptoms have been present continually for more than three months

● The patient has back stiffness on waking up in the morning

● Exercise helps to relieve the stiffness and pain

The physical exam

The doctor will assess the flexibility of a patient's spine—asking him to bend over to touch his toes, for example. The doctor may also press on the patient's sacroiliac joints to see if they are tender and measure his lung function to see if the patient has trouble inhaling completely.

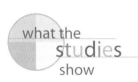

Lab-tests

Testing the patient's blood for the presence of the HLA-B27 marker can help confirm a diagnosis of AS or help rule out similar diseases like rheumatoid arthritis or lupus. But otherwise, diagnostic tests are not very useful in AS.

In studies of people with AS, the disease levelled off in almost all of them, but as many as 40 percent had restricted joint motion of the spine. Also, in the vast majority of AS sufferers, breathing ability was impaired.

X-rays

These can provide a definitive diagnosis of AS, but signs of the disease usually don't show up on an X-ray until about five years after the disease begins. The first joints to show signs of ankylosing spondylitis are usually the sacroiliac joints, which appear fuzzy on X-rays because their surfaces have been eroded by inflammation.

➡ BONING UP: Tenderness where a tendon attaches to a bone—a sharp pain in the shoulders, buttocks, back of the knees or the heel—can be a sign of early-stage ankylosing spondylitis.

What Now?

Someone recently diagnosed with AS should feel reasonably upbeat. Chances are you've been diagnosed early in the course of the disease. Today's treatments—primarily exercise and the use of NSAIDs—can almost always prevent AS from progressing to the point of irreversible spinal rigidity. These treatments also do a good job of alleviating pain and stiffness and enable most people with ankylosing spondylitis to remain active and lead normal, fulfilling lives.

Most people with AS lead normal lives, but a take-charge approach emphasizing exercise is absolutely essential for success.

The healing power of exercise. Regular activity enables AS patients to maintain a limber spine and prevent spinal deformity. Daily stretching exercises for the spine are especially recommended. Swimming may be the best overall exercise for AS patients, since it stretches the back but doesn't stress it the way running or other weight-bearing exercises do. Patients suffering from AS must also maintain as straight a spine as possible, by practicing good posture when sitting or standing and by sleeping on a firm mattress.

Drug therapy. Regular use of NSAIDs is also important in treating AS—mainly because of its effect on exercise. These anti-inflammatory drugs ease pain and stiffness enough to allow patients to engage in an active exercise program, which is critical to preventing the disease from worsening.

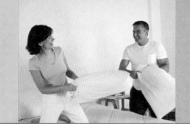
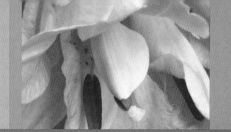

SYSTEMIC LUPUS ERYTHEMATOSUS:
the great impostor

Systemic lupus erythematosus (or simply lupus) is a chronic disease that usually inflames the joints—and also affects the skin, kidneys, blood vessels, nervous system and virtually every other organ in the body. In Canada, about 15,000 (or one in 2,000) people develop lupus, which is mainly a disease of young women. In fact, women are afflicted with lupus eight to 10 times more often than men.

What Is Lupus?

Lupus is an autoimmune disease in which the immune system produces large numbers of several different types of antibodies that attack the body's own tissues. The symptoms can vary widely, but for some people, they strongly resemble those of rheumatoid arthritis.

One common symptom is fatigue that is way out of proportion with the sufferer's activity level. Another is a persistent mild fever or a sudden flare-up of high fever. Unexplained changes in weight can also be indicators of Lupus's onset, and should be taken very seriously.

What Causes Lupus?

Experts believe people inherit a susceptibility to lupus: It is known to affect identical twins and first-degree relatives of patients are much more likely than other people to develop the disease. In lupus, the body makes antibodies that attack the nuclei and other components of its own cells.

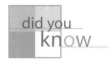

did you know

Before corticosteroids were available, the mortality rate for lupus sufferers was high. Most people with serious kidney disease died, and even those without renal disease survived in only 50 percent of the cases.

➡ **BONING UP:** Discoid lupus is limited only to the skin. Symptoms include a rash on the face, neck and scalp. This type of lupus does not affect internal organs.

Some triggering event, such as an infection or stress, may provoke lupus in genetically susceptible people. Since lupus is almost always a disease that strikes young women, hormones may also play a role in its onset.

Drug-induced lupus. Interestingly, many drugs commonly used to treat other diseases can cause temporary lupus, which disappears when the drug is stopped. Hydralazine (a high-blood-pressure medication), procainamide (used to treat irregular heartbeats) and isoniazid (a tuberculosis drug) are the chief culprits. This finding has attracted the attention of researchers who are studying how the drugs alter the immune system—findings that could shed light on how lupus develops and lead to better treatments.

How Does Lupus Progress?

Typically, a young woman will develop an array of symptoms over several months that may include worsening fatigue, weight loss, a mild fever and a great deal of joint pain that doesn't involve swelling or joint tenderness. About half of people with early lupus will also develop a butterfly-shaped facial rash that people once thought resembled a wolf's face—hence the name lupus (Latin for wolf). This distinctive rash can help in diagnosis.

Later in the course of the disease, other parts of the body may become affected, including the gastrointestinal tract (nausea, abdominal pain), blood cells (anemia), tissue surrounding the heart and lungs (inflammation) and the nervous system (headaches, seizures, strokes and hallucinations). The kidneys are an especially important target; damage to the organs can lead to kidney failure in late-stage lupus.

Other health problems that may occur in the later stages of lupus include cognitive problems, like decreased memory and difficulty doing simple math calculations. In addition, deaths from heart attack can occur due to atherosclerosis.

How Is Lupus Diagnosed?

Since it can affect so many parts of the body, lupus can mimic many diseases—making diagnosis very difficult, especially in the early stages of the condition. Presence of the butterfly rash can certainly help a doctor make the diagnosis, but a definitive diagnosis sometimes depends on two tests that detect antibodies in the blood. These antibodies—anti-nuclear antibodies and anti-DNA antibodies—both attack the nucleus of a patient's cells.

Lupus litmus tests. Virtually all lupus patients test positive on the anti-nuclear antibody (ANA) test, which makes it a very good screening test for the condition. But people who have other types of arthritis, including rheumatoid arthritis, can also test positive. So patients who are suspected of having lupus and who test positive on the ANA test, are given the anti-DNA antibody test, which is highly specific for the condition.

What Now?

Lupus can certainly be a very serious disease. On the plus side, most people with lupus can be effectively treated. Especially over the past 30 years, treatment for lupus has dramatically improved and some of the worst complications—such as kidney failure—can now almost always be avoided.

Lupus and fertility. Most people diagnosed with lupus are young women and many are concerned that the condition may impair their ability to have children. Here again the news is largely reassuring: In women severely affected by lupus, the disease may indeed impair fertility and cause more frequent miscarriages. But the great majority of women with lupus can become pregnant and have healthy babies.

Lupus and drugs. Milder forms of lupus can usually be managed with NSAIDs like ibuprofen or aspirin, which reduce inflammation and pain.

In more serious cases, when lupus affects the kidneys or other major organs, patients are usually given corticosteroids—potent anti-inflammatory drugs that can also cause serious side effects. Some two thirds of lupus patients are treated with corticosteroids.

In the most severe lupus cases, patients are treated with immunosuppressants—powerful drugs used to prevent a transplant recipient from rejecting a donated organ. They work similarly in lupus patients, by suppressing the immune system's attack on the body's organs.

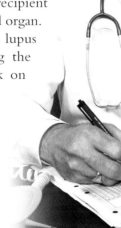

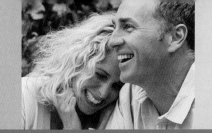
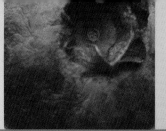
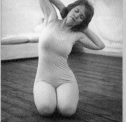

other types of arthritis

Here you will find only a small number of the types of arthritis you may be suffering from. Don't use these nutshell descriptions as a way of diagnosing your aches and pains. Make an appointment with your doctor and undergo a thorough physical. Your symptoms are unique and only your doctor can determine which disease you may have.

Finding the appropriate specialist or specialists is an important part of diagnosing your symptoms. It may take time to rule out the many other disorders that mimic your particular manifestation of arthritis before your doctor can make a final diagnosis. Once again, you and your doctor should be the architects of this important diagnosis process.

Reiter's Syndrome: It Starts with an Infection

Reiter's syndrome is a chronic, intermittent, inflammatory condition that affects not only the joints (usually starting in the knees, feet, or ankles) but also other parts of the body as well, particularly the urethra and the eyes, which can develop conjunctivitis. The syndrome is most common in men ages 20 to 40, who develop it after becoming infected with a sexually transmitted disease, though it also occurs in people with a genetic susceptibility traceable to the HLA-B27 gene.

➡ BONING UP: Reiter's syndrome is called a reactive arthritis because the joint inflammation appears to be a reaction to an infection originating in an area other than joints.

Causes and symptoms. The condition is caused by the body's abnormal response to infections (either sexually transmitted diseases or infections of the gastrointestinal tract). Symptoms include inflammation of the urethra, conjunctivitis and joint pain and inflammation—usually of the knees, toes and areas where tendons are attached to bones, such as the heels.

The combination of joint, genital, urinary, skin and eye symptoms leads a doctor to suspect Reiter's syndrome. Because these symptoms may not appear simultaneously, the disease may not be diagnosed for several months. No simple laboratory tests are available to confirm the diagnosis.

What can be done. Antibiotics are used to treat the infection and NSAIDs can minimize pain and inflammation in the joint. Although the patient often recovers, the arthritic symptoms may continue on and off for many years.

Gout: The Arthritis of Kings

Gout attacks occur when excess levels of uric acid in the

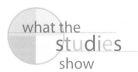

blood form needle-like crystals that typically settle in one of the joints—most commonly in the big toe but sometimes in the knee or knuckles. Once in the joint, these abrasive particles can cause excruciating pain and inflammation. The condition has afflicted royalty and the well-to-do through the ages.

Causes and symptoms. It's uncertain what precipitates a gout attack, though some factors may put you at risk. A quarter of those who suffer from gout have a family history of the illness and three-quarters have high triglyceride levels. Men who gain a lot of weight between ages 20 and 40 are particularly vulnerable. Excessive alcohol intake, high blood pressure, kidney disease, exposure to lead, crash diets and certain medications (including antibiotics, diuretics and chemotherapy drugs) may also play a role. For some people, eating foods high in chemicals called purines (such as liver or anchovies) can cause flare-ups.

Gout is diagnosed by identifying uric acid crystals in synovial fluid, usually by removing fluid from the joint through a needle. X rays can be helpful and may reveal uric acid deposits and bone damage if you have suffered from repeated inflammations.

➡ BONING UP: Drinking up to two litres of

water a day helps to incease the excretion of uric acid

What can be done. Avoiding purine-rich foods (liver and anchovies, seafoods, dried peas and beans) can help prevent gout attacks. Keeping your weight down can also help, as does avoiding foods that are high in fat and refined carbohydrates. The biggest treatment advance in managing gout is drugs like allopurinol, probenecid and sulfinpyrazone. These drugs prevent gout attacks by controlling uric acid levels in the blood. The drug colchicine, derived from the autumn crocus, is one of the oldest known remedies for gout. And a newer injectable form of the drug appears to work quickly and without side effects.

Pseudogout: Condition of the Aged

This condition is very similar to gout but is caused by different types of crystals—in this case, calcium pryophosphate dihydrate crystals, which typically form for no reason. Pseudogout is common among older people, affecting about three percent of people in their 60s and as many as half of all people over 90.

Causes and symptoms. Although the cause of pseudogout is unknown, it may occur in people who have an abnormally high calcium level in the blood, an abnormally high iron level in the tissues, or abnormally low blood levels of magnesium. Symptoms vary widely. Some people have attacks of painful arthritis, usually in the knees, wrists or other relatively large joints. Other people have lingering, chronic pain and stiffness in joints of the arms and legs, which doctors may confuse with rheumatoid arthritis. Pseudogout is diagnosed in the same manner as gout—removing fluid from the joint through a needle.

What can be done. NSAIDs are used to reduce pain and inflammation and colchicine may be given intravenously to relieve the inflammation and pain during attacks.

Polymyositis: Attack of the Muscles

Polymyositis is a chronic connective tissue disease characterized by painful inflammation and degeneration of the muscles. The condition occurs in adults from ages 40 to 60 or in children ages 5 to 15 years. Women are twice as likely as men to develop the condition.

Causes and symptoms. Although the cause is unknown, viruses or autoimmune reactions may play a role. Cancer may also trigger the disease. Symptoms, which may begin during or just after an infection, include muscle weakness (particularly in the upper arms, hips and thighs), muscle and joint pain, a rash, difficulty in swallowing, a fever, fatigue or weight loss.

Polymyositis is often diagnosed by measuring muscle weakness at the shoulders or hips, or detecting a characteristic rash or increased blood levels of certain muscle enzymes.

What can be done. Restricting activities when the inflammation is most intense often helps. Generally, an oral corticosteroid (usually prednisone) slowly improves strength and relieves pain and swelling, controlling the disease. In some cases, though, prednisone

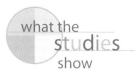
actually worsens the disease. In these cases, immunosuppressive drugs are used instead of, or alongside, prednisone.

Psoriatic Arthritis: From Skin to Joints

Psoriatic arthritis resembles rheumatoid arthritis, but doesn't produce the antibodies characteristic of RA. One negative rheumatoid factor test helps distinguish it from rheumatoid arthritis. It affects about 10 percent of people who have the skin disease psoriasis. Psoriatic arthritis may develop at any age, but typically between the ages of 30 and 50, with heredity appearing to play a significant role in susceptibility.

Causes and symptoms. Psoriasis (a skin condition causing flare-ups of red, scaly rashes and thickened, pitted nails) may precede or follow the joint inflammation. Psoriatic arthritis usually affects joints of the fingers and toes. The joints may become swollen and deformed when inflammation is chronic.

What can be done. Treatment is aimed at controlling the skin rash and alleviating the joint inflammation. Several drugs that are effective in treating rheumatoid arthritis are also used to treat psoriatic arthritis. They include gold compounds, methotrexate, cyclosporine and sulfasalazine.

Lyme Arthritis: The Biting Truth

Lyme disease is now considered a trigger for rheumatoid arthritis. The most common tick-borne disease in the United States, Lyme disease is present in southern Ontario, northeastern Manitoba, and parts of Nova Scotia, where it is carried by the deer tick, as well as southern British Columbia, where the carrier is the western blacklegged tick. The Public Health Agency of Canada states that these ticks are sometimes carried to other parts of Canada by migratory birds, and that they can also be active during the winter months in regions where the wintertime temperatures hover at around 4°C.

It is important to bear in mind, however, that Lyme disease is not actually a very common ailment in Canada or in many other parts of the world.

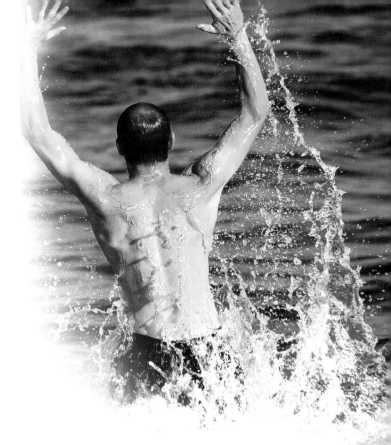

Causes and symptoms. People become infected when bitten by ticks that carry Lyme bacteria (known as *Borrellia burgdoferi*). Early Lyme disease symptoms include a ring-like rash at the point of initial infection and flu-like symptoms such as fatigue, fever, chills and headache. If you are suffering the general symptoms listed above and have recently been in a Lyme hot zone, it's advisable to request a blood test that specifically looks for Lyme disease.

Prompt treatment with antibiotics can cure the infection. But without treatment, about 50 percent of infected people experience intermittent arthritis in various joints. The arthritis usually clears up on its own, but about 10 percent of people develop chronic inflammatory arthritis, most often in the knee.

What can be done. The best strategy is to avoid tick bites. People who go outside in Lyme-disease areas should wear light-coloured clothes (so ticks will be visible), tuck pant cuffs into socks (to keep ticks away from the skin), use repellents containing the ingredient DEET and conduct daily tick checks to remove ticks before they can bite. The Public Health Agency of Canada states that treatment for those already infected with Lyme disease calls for treatments of doxycycline, ceftriaxone or amoxicillin.

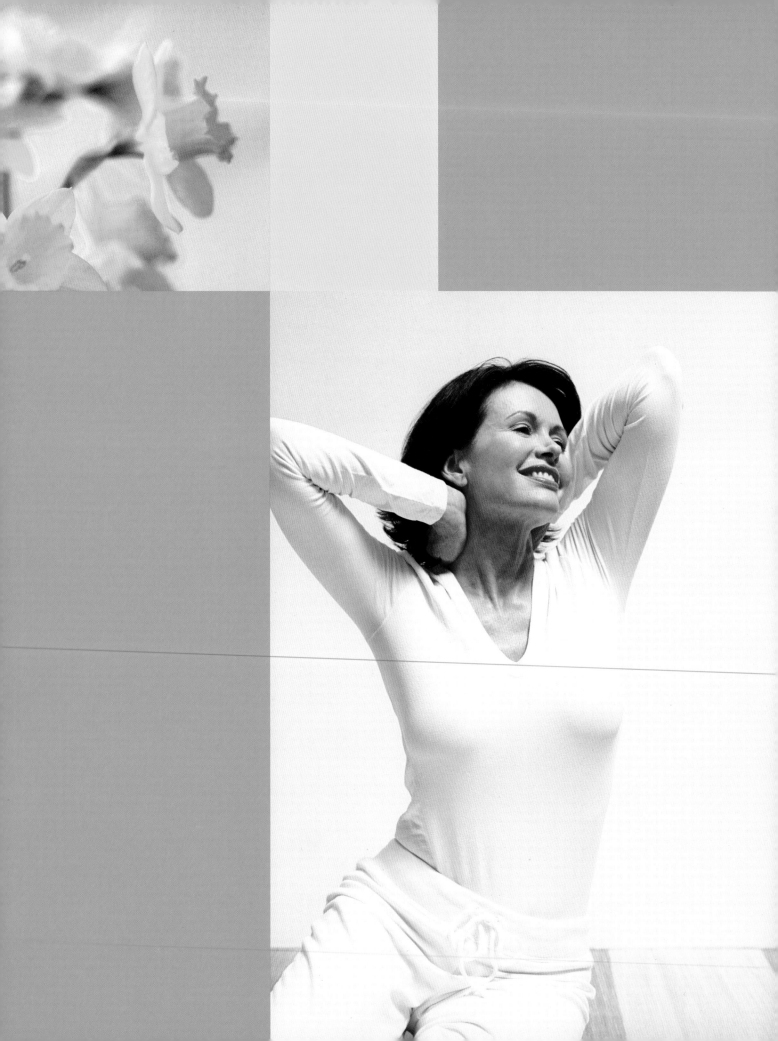

you can beat arthritis

When you have arthritis, it's easy to let scary words like

"degenerative" and "progressive" become stumbling blocks—

as if there's nothing you can do to ease your pain and stay

functional. In fact, this is far from the truth. Though arthritis is

degenerative by nature, there is plenty you can do to slow its

progress—or even halt it altogether. Exercise and a healthy

diet top the list of steps you can take, but they'll be even more

effective as part of a comprehensive self-care program that

uses all the comfort-keeping methods you can muster.

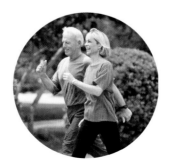

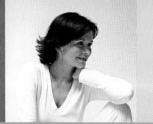

the arthritis action plan

Acute health problems are different from chronic ones. Acute health problems appear abruptly and don't last long: They typically either get better on their own (like food poisoning, colds, or bruises) or respond promptly to treatment (surgery to remove an inflamed appendix, penicillin to kill strep throat bacteria).

Chronic illnesses usually develop slowly and then linger—"chronic," by definition, means you have a problem indefinitely or even for life. And although acute health problems usually run a predictable course of illness followed by healing and cure, a diagnosis of arthritis involves uncertainty and many questions:

● Will I have to give up my favourite activities?

● Can therapies keep my disease from progressing?

● Will additional joints become affected?

● Can I continue to provide for my family?

● Can I perform the simple activities of everyday life that allow me to stay independent?

● How can I deal with anger and frustration?

● How will this affect my relationships?

➡ BONING UP: Always use the strongest, largest joints and muscles for a given job. Getting up from a chair places a great deal of strain on your hands if you push yourself with your fingertips. Instead of using your fingers or knuckles, use your palms to help you achieve liftoff.

Patient in Charge

For people with chronic health problems, every single day presents a series of complex challenges. Even as they cope with their specific condition medically and surgically, these people face tremendous uncertainty regarding the course of their disease and its impact on their lives. Add all these burdens to the pain and disability caused by the chronic illness itself and patients can become frustrated and depressed.

Clearly, the key ingredient in managing a chronic condition is the patient's own involvement in making the decisions about his or her care.

Passive to aggressive. This need for patients to participate in their own health care may seem obvious now. But until recently, most patients with chronic health problems took a back-seat approach to treatment. They went to the doctor to find out how they were doing and rarely asked questions. If a drug wasn't helping or was causing adverse effects, they would rarely complain: After all, who were they to question the doctor's wisdom or to judge whether a treatment was working?

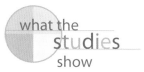

When patients with chronic health problems—hypertension, diabetes and peptic ulcers— were coached on how to become more assertive with their doctors, they reported better overall health and fewer limitations on their social and work lives due to illness.

THE COURSE THAT CHANGES LIVES

In follow-up studies involving people enrolled in arthritis self-management courses, researchers found that the positive attitude gained by participants is crucial for reducing pain and disability. The studies also produced a number of other intriguing results, including:

1. Twenty months after completing the course, participants on average had reduced their pain by 20 percent, their depression by 14 percent and visits to physicians by 35 percent compared with their situation before enrolling.

2. The beneficial effects from participating in the course lasted. Four years after taking the course, patients noted that pain levels were 19 percent lower and doctor visits had been reduced by 43 percent than before enrolling in the course.

3. Those who fail to benefit from arthritis self-management courses tend to be fatalistic people who believe that nothing can be done about their arthritis.

Accentuate the Positive

You are probably familiar with Norman Vincent Peale's book, *The Power of Positive Thinking*. The take-charge approach emphasizes something similar: the power of a positive attitude. Studies have shown that when people adopt a take-charge attitude toward their arthritis, this itself can do wonders for their pain and disability.

Stay the course. This approach was emphasized in the Arthritis Self-Management Program developed by Stanford University in 1979. The US Arthritis Foundation adopted the program in 1984 for its arthritis self-help course. And the Arthritis Society has helped literally thousands of Canadian arthritis sufferers with its Arthritis Self-Management Program. And we're not alone; many countries have used the Stanford-developed program as the basis for their own arthritis self-help programs.

Numerous studies have evaluated the success of self-management courses in improving the health of arthritis patients. In doing their follow-up studies, researchers had expected that the behaviours taught in the course—exercising more and eating healthier, for example—would have the biggest impact on improving participants' health. But the experts made a surprising finding.

Learned optimism. Participants had indeed changed their behaviour for the better after taking the course and they experienced significantly less pain and disability compared with patients who hadn't enrolled. But their improved health did not flow primarily from the behaviour changes they'd made. Instead, the researchers found, participants' success in regaining their health hinged mainly on something else they got from the course: the confidence that they were able to control their arthritis symptoms.

A take-charge attitude, it turns out, can be learned—and is the key ingredient for over-coming arthritis.

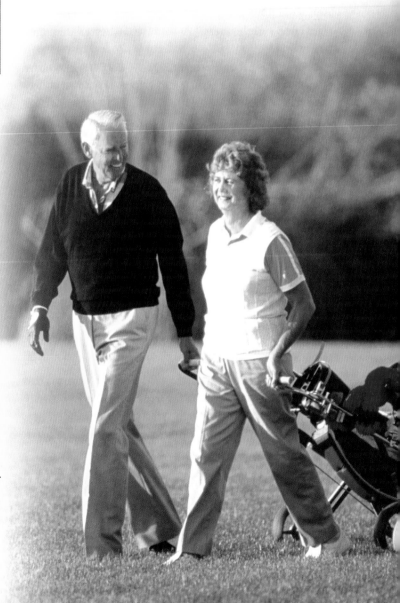

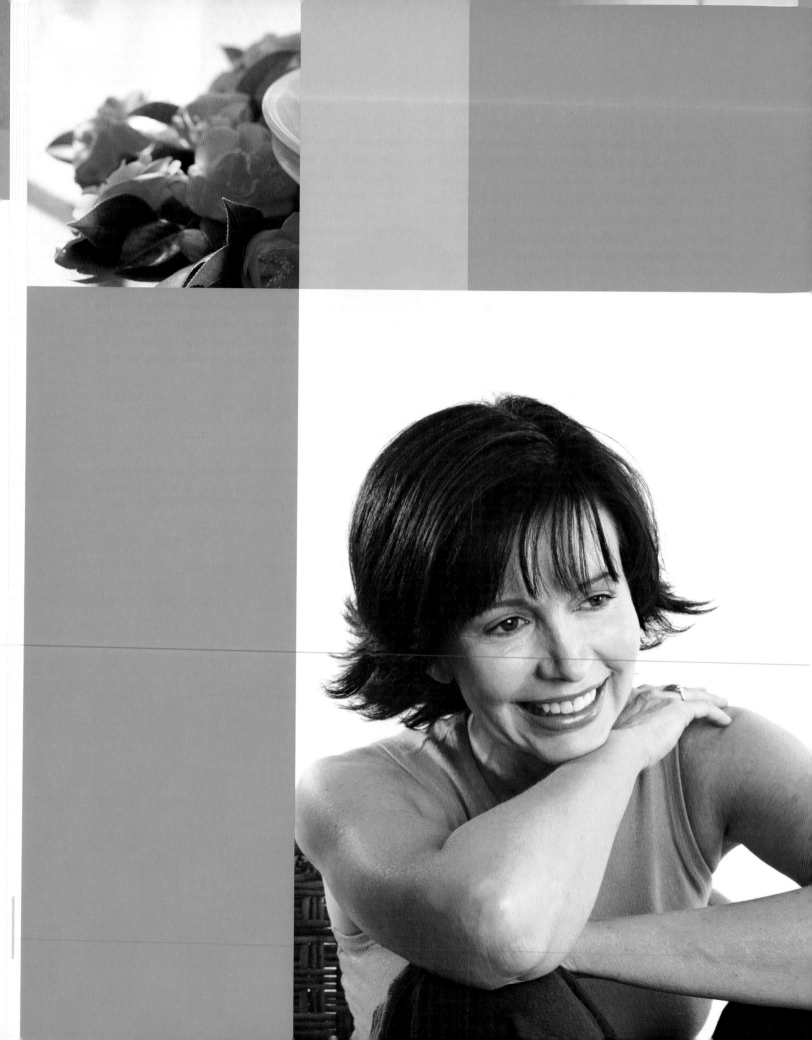

targeted exercises

The pages ahead may seem intimidating, even frightening. All these exercises! So much instruction! If this was your reaction, it's time for a change of attitude. Think of this part as a cookbook: a wonderful array of healthy movements to browse and sample, none mandatory but all good for you. ● When you look closely, you'll discover that these stretches, exercises and massages are simple, gentle and natural—perfect for people with arthritis! So give them a try. Then, in Part Four, we'll show you how to put them together into the perfect regular routine.

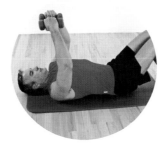

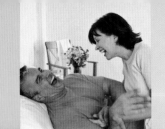
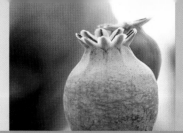

getting into action

Think of Part One of this book as "ready," and Part Two as "set." Now you're at "go!" In the pages ahead, you will discover a broad range of stretches, strengthening moves and massages, most of them quite unlike what you would find in more general fitness books. The differences? First, they are gentler and more natural movements. Second, they were chosen as much for their beneficial effects for joints as for their effectiveness in building muscle.

Maybe you already do simple range-of-motion exercises or take strolls around your neighbourhood fairly regularly. That puts you ahead of the game. What happens next is not a race, but a journey. There's nobody to beat and you don't have to push yourself too hard. Comfortable, week-by-week progress will move you toward your beginning goals. Then you'll be able to establish new goals that you could not even have imagined at the start.

The exercises in this section are the key to your success in fighting pain and getting fit. Each is explained step by step, with plenty of tips and secrets from some of the best experts on making exercise work for people with arthritis. Not every exercise will be right for you. Start by establishing your level of physical function using the self-scoring questions (next page). If you already know at which level you should begin, use the reminder chart "Figuring Your Function Level" to establish the starting parameters for your program. Keep in mind that these guidelines are starting points and are deliberately on the conservative side. The last thing you need is an exercise program that causes more pain. But even after one or two workouts, you'll have a sense of whether you can handle more. If you're comfortable taking on harder exercises without causing significant discomfort, feel free to do more repetitions, stretch longer, choose more challenging movements or add time to your cardio workout.

Once you get started with a program, you'll quickly become comfortable with the motions your exercises require. In many cases, it's possible for simple modifications to make the exercises you're doing more challenging as you get more fit, so you don't have to change a routine you already like. At the same time, if you want to move on to new exercises or add elements to your workout, you'll find options for doing so.

The Parts and the Whole

Bodybuilders and serious fitness enthusiasts love to talk about "isolating" muscles—doing exercises that concentrate on a single muscle that will produce just the right ripple to enhance the exerciser's buff beauty. Your goals are more pragmatic. When you strive to improve function, isolating muscles can indeed build strength in critical areas that support arthritic joints. But it's just as important to make muscles work together. That, after all, is how the body operates in real life.

Physiologists think of the body as a mechanical system of many segments in which forces applied to one joint can cause a chain reaction of effects in other joints through the levers of the skeleton and the muscles. (They call it the kinetic chain.) Sometimes these effects can be predicted. For example, if you have arthritis in one knee, the way you move your body to compensate raises your risk of arthritis in the opposite knee and hip.

Bottom line: Physiologists say that in addition to exercises that work specific muscles, it's important to do exercises or activities that work bones, joints and muscles in ways they actually function in day-to-day activities such as climbing stairs or getting out of a chair. And if you have arthritis in the knee, don't just work to strengthen muscles supporting that joint, but build strength throughout the rest of your body as well. "Everything is connected to everything else," says Virginia Kraus, M.D., Ph.D., medical director of the Arthritis Rehabilitation Program at Duke University Center for Living. "So it's important to do a variety of exercises, such as aerobic walking in addition to a range of strength exercises."

That's an important message. While the pages ahead are organized by the joints of the body, don't limit yourself to the exercises targeted at your problem spot. Indeed, as important as it is to learn these exercises properly, it is just as important to learn how to put them together into a sequence that is absolutely best for you and your needs. That is what Part Four is all about. By using these two sections together, you have the ultimate resource for exercising away arthritis pain.

FIGURING YOUR FUNCTION LEVEL

Whatever your level of function, you'll find exercises in this section that you can do without causing further pain. Follow the guidelines below to decide which exercises are appropriate for your function level. To determine what level you should start with, take the self-scoring quiz on this page. And don't forget to make aerobic exercise a part of your routine!

LEVEL 1

Low Physical Function

- **Flexibility:** Hold stretches for 15 seconds
- **Strength:** 1 set of 6 repetitions with an easy weight, two to three days a week
- **Aerobics:** 5 minutes a day, three to five days a week

LEVEL 2

Moderate Physical Function

- **Flexibility:** Hold stretches for 20 seconds
- **Strength:** 1 set of 6 to 8 repetitions with an easy weight, two to three days a week
- **Aerobics:** 10 to 12 minutes a day, three to five days a week

LEVEL 3

Good Physical Function

- **Flexibility:** Hold stretches for 30 seconds
- **Strength:** 1 set of 8 repetitions with a moderate weight, two to three days a week
- **Aerobics:** 20 minutes a day, three to five days a week

Modifying Your Program

Everybody has good days and bad. But some bad days are worse than others. How should you change—not abandon—your exercise program in response to flare-ups of pain or the draggy torpor of fatigue? Score your responses to the following questions and adjust your program as suggested below.

How much pain do you have today?

NONE	0
VERY MILD	1
MILD	2
MODERATE	3
SEVERE	4
WORST	5

How much fatigue do you have today?

NONE	0
VERY MILD	1
MILD	2
MODERATE	3
SEVERE	4
WORST	5

Scoring

With pain or fatigue scores of:

0–2 Proceed as planned with your exercise program, gradually increasing intensity as improvements in your fitness and function allow.

3 Exercise at the same level as the previous session (without adding resistance or intensity), if you exercised within the past week.

4 Reduce the number of repetitions of strength exercises and aerobic time by 50 percent.

5 It may be best not to do your regular exercise routine today. But try to do some simple, gentle body movements throughout the day, perhaps after taking a warm bath or shower.

The knees and hips are the body's main weight-bearing joints, subject to enormous stress from daily activities. Just stepping up a single stair, for example, puts hundreds of pounds of pressure on lower-body joints and the muscles that support them. You can't do much to make your joints more durable, but making your muscles stronger lets them take on more of the load, relieving your knees and hips.

"Muscles of hips and knees are critical for mobility and everyday function, whether you're taking the stairs, getting out of a car or lifting laundry or groceries," says Daniel Rooks, Ph.D., director of the Tanger Be Well Center for Health Management at Harvard's Beth Israel Deaconess Medical Center. "They often work together, so you want a mix of exercises that strengthen multiple muscles together along with exercises that work muscles supporting the joints separately."

STRETCHES

Wall Sit

This is a gentle move to stretch stiff hamstrings at the back of the leg.

1. Sit on the floor, back against a wall, knees bent and heels, hip-width apart, planted two feet in front of you. Your toes should point upward at a 45-degree angle.

2. Slowly slide or walk your heels forward so that your knees get closer to the ground until you feel a slight stretch at the back of your knees **a**. Relax your muscles and hold this position.

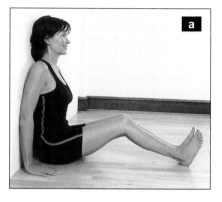

TIP: Pressing your back against the wall keeps your pelvis fixed so that all movement is concentrated on your hamstrings.

Seated Knee Extension

This is a good stretch and warmup for a strength exercise, since it uses the same basic motion with weights. You need a chair high enough to slightly elevate your heels off the floor. To give a regular chair extra height, use cushions.

1. Sit in a chair, back straight, both feet flat on the floor and knees bent 90 degrees.

2. Slowly straighten your right knee as far as you comfortably can, so that toes point toward the ceiling **a**. Hold. Repeat with the other leg.

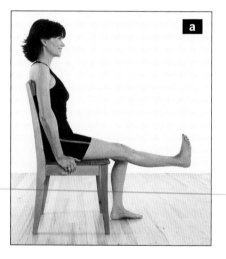

TIP: Keep your spine pressed against the back of the chair so that you don't arch your back. If the quadriceps muscles at the front of your thighs are weak, this movement will help strengthen them while also stretching your hamstrings.

Straight-Leg Stretch

If you can sit and straighten your legs in front of you, try this more advanced stretch.

1. Sit on the floor, legs extended straight in front of you, toes pointed toward the ceiling. Keep your back straight and your hands on the outside of your thighs.

2. Slide your hands forward along your legs toward your toes, reaching as far as you comfortably can and putting your chest as close to your knees as possible **a**. Hold for a gentle stretch at the back of your legs.

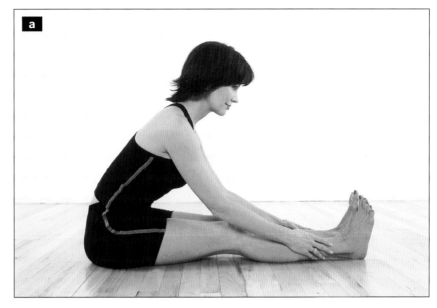

TIP: Don't arch your back during the stretch: A straight spine protects the back and allows a better stretch of your hamstrings. You don't have to reach your toes: As you become more limber, you'll be able to reach farther.

Seated V

This exercise lengthens the adductor muscles of the groin area in the inner thigh as well as the hamstrings—a twist allows you to stretch both sets of muscles.

1. Sit on the floor, back straight, legs extended, toes pointed toward the ceiling and feet spread comfortably apart in a V. Hands should rest in front of you between your thighs **a**.

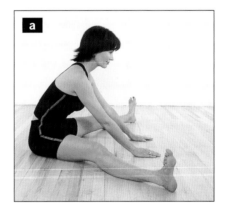

2. Keeping your back straight, gently "walk" your hands out in front of you until you feel a slight stretch in your inner thighs **b**. Hold.

TIP: Use this position for a hamstring stretch by putting your left hand on the inside of your right thigh and the right hand on the outside, then moving both hands down your right leg. Hold and repeat on the left leg.

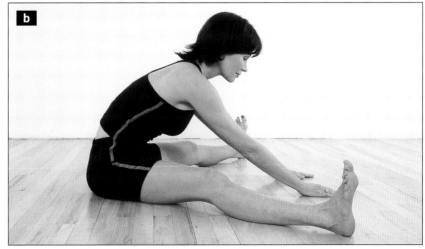

Standing Quad Stretch

Top athletes use this stretch for lengthening the all-important quadriceps muscle on the front of the thigh.

1. Stand with feet about hip-width apart, holding on to a chair or counter with your left hand.

2. Standing on your left leg with the knee slightly flexed, bend your right knee so that your foot is behind you. Keeping your knees next to each other, gently bring your right heel toward your buttocks.

Grab your right foot with your right hand **a**. Hold.

3. Let your right foot down and repeat with your left leg.

TIP: Keep your knees close together during the stretch. If muscles are tight, you'll tend to move at the hip rather than the knee, which changes the stretch. If you have trouble balancing or experience pain standing on one leg, you can perform this same move while lying on your stomach.

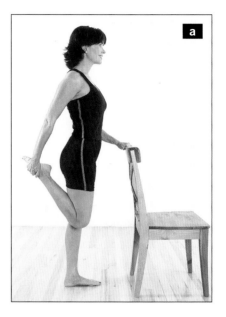

Lying Quad and Hip Stretch

Similar to the standing quad stretch, this exercise works both the quadriceps and the hip flexor muscles, prime movers in the torso.

1. Lie on your left side, using your left arm as a pillow to support your head. Bend your left hip (which is resting on the floor) to a 90-degree angle so that your knee is in front of you **a**.

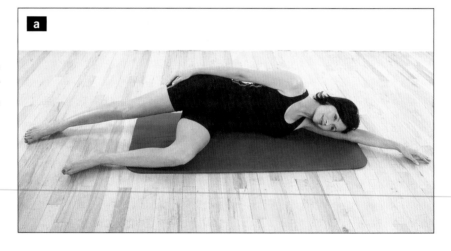

2. Bend your top (right) knee to a 90-degree angle, grabbing your right ankle with your right hand and bringing the heel back toward the buttocks **b**. Hold. Repeat with the other leg.

TIP: Don't straighten your bottom knee. Keeping the knee bent helps fix the pelvis in a slightly forward position that provides a better hip stretch when you move the top leg back.

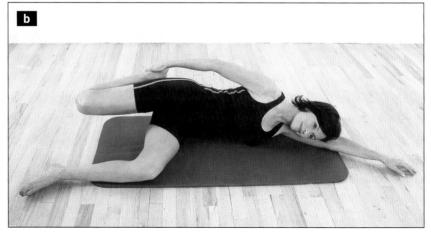

Lying Pelvis Rotation

This simple move uses gravity to stretch the abductor muscles on the outside of the hip.

1. Lie on your right side, using your right arm as a pillow to support your head. Keeping your right leg straight, bend your left hip at a 90-degree angle so your knee is in front of you.

2. Relax the muscles of your left leg so that your left knee slowly drops toward the ground to produce a gentle rotational stretch of the hip **a**. Stay relaxed and hold. Repeat with the other leg.

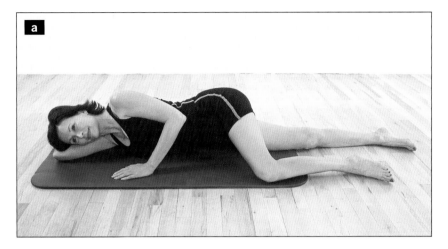

TIP: Start with the lying pelvis rotation if your hip muscles are tight. When you're more limber, try a variation: Lie on your back with feet flat on floor so your knees are pointing toward the ceiling. Keeping shoulders on the ground, slowly lower both knees to the right to get a stretch in left hip and buttocks. Hold, return to the starting position and repeat on the other side.

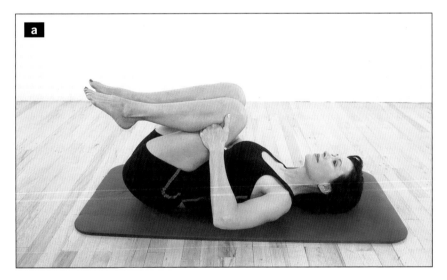

Knees to Chest

A classic for easing low back discomfort, this stretch can be done lying on a bed and also helps your hips and knees.

1. Lie on your back with legs relaxed and straight, toes pointing toward the ceiling.

2. Put your hands on the back of your thighs under your knees and smoothly pull both knees as far toward your shoulders as is comfortable to stretch the extensor muscles at the back of the hips in the buttocks area **a**. Hold.

everyday secrets

Wide-ranging advice for better fitness, more movement and safer exercise for people with arthritis.

Keep eyes open. You may be tempted to close your eyes during exercise so you can concentrate on your muscles or breathing. Don't. Balance relies on visual input to the brain; keep your eyes open to steady yourself.

Spread correctly. Many exercise guides tell you to start standing exercises with your feet shoulder-width apart. If you have arthritis, plant your feet hip-width apart. This narrower distance puts your knees, hips and feet in alignment for good posture and improved biomechanics.

Keep support nearby. During standing exercises, use—or keep within easy grasp—a sturdy chair, countertop or even wall, to maintain your balance and reduce the risk of injury.

Build abs with reps. The abdominal exercises in this book don't use weights, so when you master the most difficult version of a given exercise, how do you top that? Try to add a repetition at least every other time you do the exercise.

continued on page 64

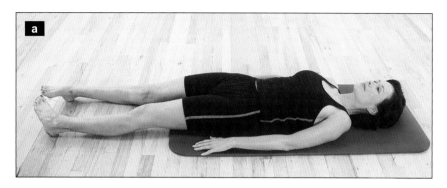

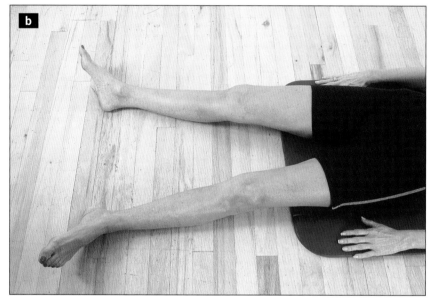

Leg Twist

Another comfortable stretch that can be done in bed, this windshield wiper motion stretches the hip rotator muscles, which helps hip mobility and may help ease pain from sciatica.

1. Lie on your back with feet about shoulder-width apart, toes pointed toward the ceiling.

2. Smoothly rotate your ankles to first roll your toes toward each other **a**. Hold. Now rotate ankles to roll toes away from each other **b**. Hold.

TIP: You don't have to be lying down to do this stretch. Performed while sitting on the floor, it's particularly effective when done from the seated V position.

STRENGTH EXERCISES

LEVEL 1

Partial Squat

Squats build strength on all sides of your upper legs and buttocks, supporting a wide variety of everyday activities. If you experience knee pain, start with this mild version.

1. Stand with feet about hip-width apart, touching a chair or counter for balance.

2. Keeping your back straight and your eyes looking forward, slowly lower your body as if you were going to sit in a chair **a** . Stop when you reach a point halfway to a sitting position, then raise yourself back to a standing position.

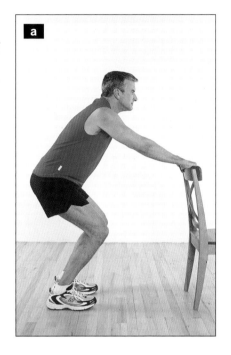

TIP: Your legs should do the work. Use the chair or countertop only to keep your balance, not to support your weight. Try to do the exercise hands-free. To keep your body properly aligned, think about pushing down with your heels. Don't let your knees move forward of your toes.

NOTCH IT UP: Lower yourself all the way to a chair. From the same starting position, sit lightly on the front half of a chair, then immediately stand up again.

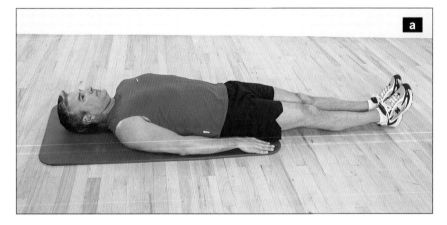

Lying Hip Abduction

Like the leg part of making snow angels (only you're warm and dry), this exercise works the abductor muscles at the outside of the hip.

1. Lie on your back with your feet pointing toward the ceiling and your legs together **a** .

2. Keeping your legs straight, move your feet comfortably apart and bring them back together again **b** .

TIP: Do this gently and slowly, pausing at the full extension. A fast scissoring motion isn't as safe or as beneficial for your muscles.

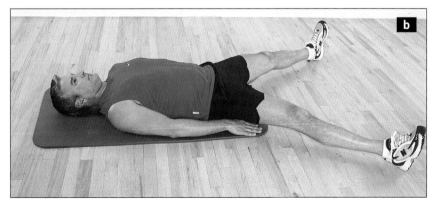

Knees and Hips >

Heel Slide

This simple exercise with two vari-ations works the hamstring muscles.

1. Lie on your back with your legs straight and your toes pointed toward the ceiling **a**.

2. Keeping your left leg straight, slowly bend your right leg so your knee moves toward the ceiling and your heel slides toward your buttocks **b**.

3. Slide your heel back to the starting position. After one set, repeat with the other leg.

NOTCH IT UP: Start by doing one leg at a time. As you gain strength, do both legs together, which is more difficult.

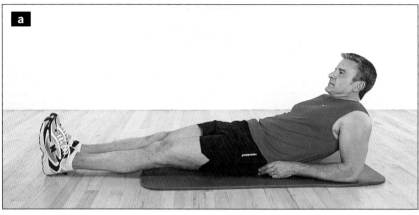

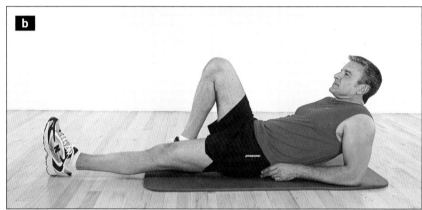

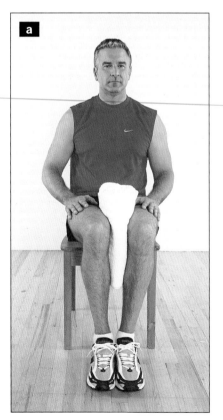

Towel Squeeze

This is an isometric exercise that safely works the muscles of the inner thigh, which help stabilize the knees and hips.

1. Sit in a chair with a large, rolled-up bath towel placed between your knees and thighs.

2. Gently squeeze your knees to-gether as firmly as you comfortably can **a**. Hold for six seconds to do one repetition.

TIP: Don't worry if your knees touch as long as the contact doesn't cause pain: The towel is meant to cushion knees, not separate them. If you prefer, you can also use a folded bed pillow or a small sofa pillow.

Lower-Body Extension

Though this exercise by itself provides a good workout for the hips, a more advanced version in level 2, the Bird Dog, offers a combined move that also targets the upper body.

1. Get down on your hands and knees on the floor, a rug or an exercise mat.

2. Extend your right leg out behind you, keeping your foot about one inch off the floor as you straighten your knee **a** . Return to the starting position and repeat with the other leg to complete one repetition. Continue alternating legs until you finish a set.

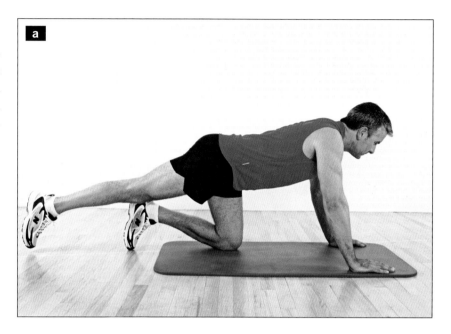

Lying Hip Extension

This exercise works large muscles in the hips and buttocks as well as the hamstrings, which stabilize the hips and help walking and sitting.

1. Lie on your stomach with your legs straight and your toes pointed down. You can prop your upper body on your elbows, but may find it more relaxing to lie flat, supporting your head with your arms or hands.

2. Keeping your knee straight, lift your entire right leg so that your foot is 1 to 2 inches (2.5 to 5 cm) off the floor **a** . Lower your leg back to the floor.

3. Repeat with the other leg. This is one repetition.

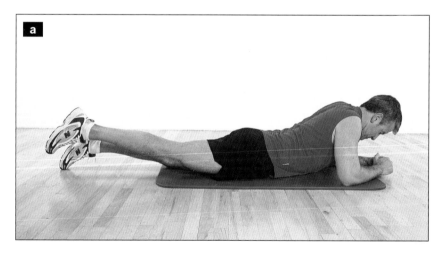

TIP: Keep your body stable and relaxed so that all movement is concentrated at the hip joint.

NOTCH IT UP: As you become stronger, you can make this exercise more intense by doing extra repetitions or adding strap-on ankle weights.

Knees and Hips >

everyday secrets

Know which side. If pain or decreased range of motion makes walking difficult, use a cane or rolling walker in the hand opposite the painful knee or hip.

Consider a splint. If overzealous exercising makes joint pain flare up, give the injured area a rest. A splint will temporarily stabilize the joint and keep you from hurting it further. You can buy splints over the counter at a drugstore or get them fitted by an occupational therapist. You can buy splints for fingers, hands, wrists, elbows, knees and ankles.

Know the limits. If you've had total hip or knee replacement, check with your doctor before doing any exercises. These procedures eliminate certain moves from your repertoire for at least two to six months after surgery. You should, for example, avoid exercises that involve high-impact stress on the lower extremities, leg adduction (moving legs inward against resistance) or flexing the new joint beyond 90 degrees.

continued on page 68

LEVEL 2

Standing Hip Extension

A standing version of the lying hip extension in level 1 (page 63), this exercise provides a more intense workout for the hips, buttocks, hamstrings and lower back.

1. Stand with feet about hip-width apart, lightly holding a chair or counter.

2. Without bending the knee, move your right leg from the hip back behind you **a**. Return slowly to the starting position. After one set, repeat with the other leg.

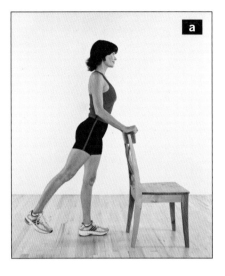

TIPS: Don't lock the knee of the leg you stand on, but instead keep it slightly bent. While the motion is pendulum-like, you shouldn't let momentum do the work. Perform the move slowly, especially during the return phase.

Standing Knee Flexion

A tandem exercise to the seated knee extension (page 56), this move strengthens the hamstrings at the back of the thigh.

1. Wearing ankle weights, stand behind a chair with feet about hip-width apart, holding on to the back of the chair.

2. Smoothly bend your left knee, drawing your heel toward your buttocks **a**, then slowly return your foot to the ground. After one set, repeat with the other leg.

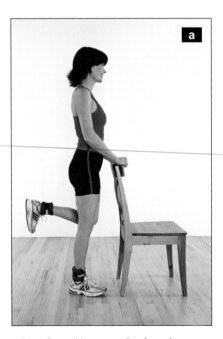

TIPS:
• Start with enough weight to allow you to comfortably do the 6 to 8 repetitions suggested for level 2 exercises.

• Keep your knees next to each other as you bend your knee so that your upper legs remain parallel.

• Start by raising your heel so that your lower leg is parallel to the floor. As you become more conditioned, lift your heel closer to your buttocks. Add weight as you gain strength.

Side Hip Abduction

This simple exercise works the abductor muscles on the outside of the hip and outer thigh.

1. Lie on your left side with both legs extended and resting one on top of the other, supporting your head with your left hand.

2. In a smooth and controlled motion, lift your fully extended right leg straight up as high as you comfortably can **a**. Then lower it back to the starting position. After one set, repeat with the other leg.

TIP: If you feel unstable in the starting position, try bending the lower leg to provide a wider base of support.

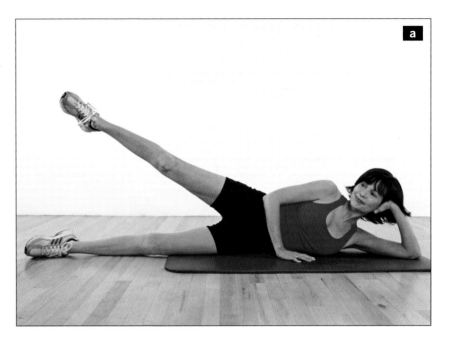

Stair Step-Up

Easily a part of any exercise routine, the step-up can be modified in a variety of ways to make it more challenging as you progress.

1. Stand in front of a step with both feet on the floor about hip-width apart.

2. Place your right foot solidly on the stair and step up **a**. Bring your left foot up and touch it lightly on the step before lowering it back to the floor **b**.

3. Step down with your right foot.

4. Step up with your left foot, bringing your right foot up and touching it lightly on the step, then lowering it back to the floor. Alternate steps in this way, counting one repetition when each foot has stepped up one time.

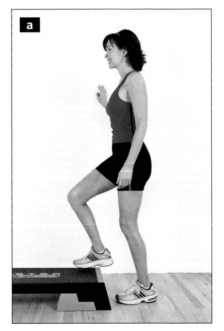

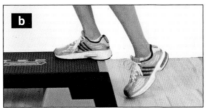

TIP: To keep track of repetitions, count step-ups on just one foot. Though you can use a special exercise step for this move, it's not necessary. In fact, a regular step in your home may be preferable because you can lightly grasp the stair rail for support.

NOTCH IT UP: The first way to make this exercise more difficult is to do a set using only one foot instead of alternating. For example, use the right foot to step up, step down, then step up again rather than alternating with the left foot. When you've finished a set of step-ups with the right foot, do a set with the left. A second way to make this exercise more difficult is to alternate your feet, but raise yourself up two steps at a time instead of just one.

everyday
secrets

Use good gear. Theoretically, anything heavy can be used for resistance exercises—milk jugs filled with sand or bags of rice. Such ad hoc gear may keep your equipment costs down, but most resistance exercises are more effective, more comfortable and safer if you use equipment designed for fitness use.

Do it softly and twice. If you find a particular stretch difficult, don't push it. Instead, do the stretch as well as you can twice, resting in between. The repeated lengthening of your muscles will provide an extra degree of flexibility.

Add sets, not weights. A more intense exercise is usually taken to mean one involving heavier weights. But the issue is the overall volume of exercise, not just the weight of resistance. If you want to make an exercise more intense but find additional resistance to be uncomfortable, you can add sets or repetitions for an extra challenge.

continued on page 76

Partial Stationary Lunge

The lunge is a time-tested exercise that really builds up the muscles involved with walking, climbing stairs and getting out of a chair.

1. Take a larger-than-normal step forward with your right foot. This is your starting position and you'll keep both feet planted through your repetitions **a**.

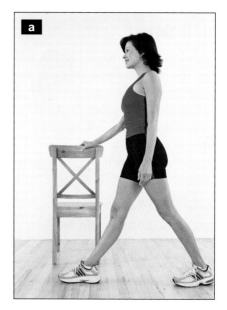

2. Keeping your upper body straight, bend your right knee and slide your pelvis forward until your knee is over the toe of your right foot **b**. The heel of your left foot will come off the floor. To further lower your body, bend your left knee.

3. Return to the starting position and repeat on the same side. After one set, do the same with the other leg.

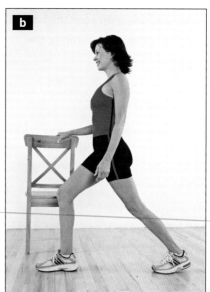

TIP: The difficulty of this move can be adjusted by the size of your starting step: Every increase of distance intensifies resistance. When you can do 12 repetitions comfortably, extend your first step another half foot (15 cm). If needed, use a chair or counter to keep your balance, but not to support your weight.

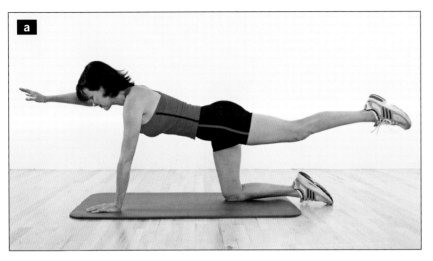

Advanced Bird Dog

Building on the basic bird dog move in level 2, this more advanced exercise not only works muscles of the hips, but also the back and shoulders.

1. Get down on your hands and knees on the floor, a rug or an exercise mat.

2. Extend your left leg out behind you, raising your foot so that your entire leg is parallel to the floor—a more strenuous position than in the basic bird dog. At the same time, reach out straight in front of you with your right arm **a**.

3. Return to the starting position and repeat with the other leg and arm to complete one repetition. Continue alternating legs and arms until you finish a set.

AT THE *Fitness Centre*

If you have access to good-quality exercise machines, here's what to use for your knees and hips:

LEG PRESS

There are many types of leg-press machines, but with the best units for people with arthritis, extending your legs during the lift moves the seat, not the foot plate. This prevents uneven or sudden pressure on knees if you perform the exercise too quickly. With machines that move the foot plate, you must keep movements slow and controlled. Machines with reclining seats in which your body forms a V are most comfortable. Machines in which you lie flat with feet directly overhead are difficult to get in and out of.

KNEE EXTENSION

You have unlimited resistance variations with a machine to do this exercise for your quadriceps. Although this exercise can be done one leg at a time (especially during rehabilitation), doing both legs at once promotes muscle balance by encouraging both sides of the body to work together like they do in daily life.

KNEE FLEXION

This is often a tandem exercise with the knee extension, designed to work your hamstrings. You may find older versions of this machine in which you do the exercise lying down. These machines work well, but you'll find a seated machine easier to mount and dismount.

MACHINE ABDUCTION/ ADDUCTION

Machines are a great way to isolate the muscles at the sides of your upper leg. If your gym doesn't have a single machine that does both abduction and adduction, it should have separate machines for doing these same movements. When beginning with a machine, use the same resistance for both abduction and adduction.

Knees and Hips >

MASSAGES

Hip Circle

This gentle massage helps boost circulation in the hip.

1. Before you start, place your hands on your hips and hold for a moment, then begin rubbing your palms over the sides of your hips in large circles to improve circulation close to the surface of the skin **a**.

2. Resting your thumb on your waist for support, use your fingers to press firmly on the side of your hip **b**. Move your fingers in a circular motion to stimulate blood flow deeper in the muscle.

Kneecap Squeeze

This massage expels fluid from the knee joint when you squeeze, but allows it to flow back more abundantly when you release, giving some relief from pain.

1. Sit in a chair and place your right hand over your right knee so that your palm is covering your kneecap.

2. Use your fingers and thumb to squeeze the sides of your kneecap **a**. Hold the squeeze for about two seconds, then release. Repeat on the left knee.

Knee Orbit

A thorough workover relaxes the knee joint.

1. Sit in a chair and place your right hand over your right knee. Find the edge of your kneecap with your fingers, then gently massage with small, circular motions **a**.

2. Continue massaging as you move your fingers around the entire perimeter of the kneecap **b**. Include the top area where thigh muscles attach to the kneecap **c**. Continue the massage for one to two minutes, then repeat on the left knee.

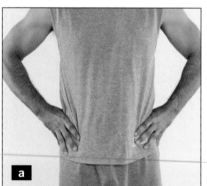

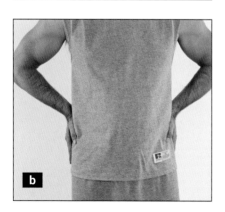

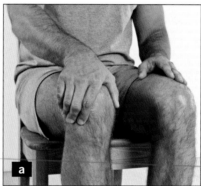

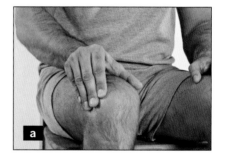

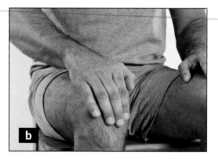

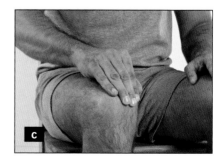

12 WAYS TO WALK MORE

You exercise your hips and knees so you can walk more, without pain or exhaustion. But doctors will also tell you that the best way to walk more is to … walk more. Here are 12 ideas to get you on your feet and moving:

1. Every night, immediately after dinner, take a 20-minute stroll. Don't let the weather stop you—that's what jackets, boots and umbrellas are for. In fact, there's something wonderfully refreshing and childlike about a walk in the rain or snow. After dinner is the perfect time for a walk. It gets you away from the television, it's when others are outside, it's a lovely time of day and it stops you from eating more.

2. Develop a habit: Never sit while talking on the phone. Instead, walk around your home if you have a portable phone and if not, pace back and forth. You'd be surprised how much movement you can do when you are concentrating on a conversation rather than the exertion.

3. Make more social events around walking. For example, rather than meeting friends for coffee or lunch, suggest meeting at the public gardens for a stroll.

4. When watching television, always get up and move about during commercials. You've seen them already, anyhow. During a single one-hour show, you can get in more than 10 minutes of activity!

5. Take the stairs, take the stairs, take the stairs. You've heard it a million times, but if it is three flights or less, you have no excuse to take an elevator, unless your arthritis pain is truly prohibitive. In that case, take one flight of stairs instead.

6. For an evening's diversion, do some outdoor window-shopping. Strolling down a street of shops is great for people-watching, talking and feeling alive.

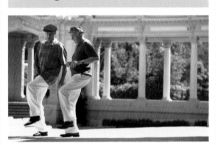

7. Split your lunch hour in two: 30 minutes of eating, 30 minutes of walking. No one needs to eat for 60 minutes. Chances are, you're just sitting and talking. Invite your lunch partner along for the stroll.

8. Find a park or a wilderness area near you and commit to a nature walk a few times a week. Nothing lifts your soul as much as a good walk in the woods (or by the lake or even in the desert).

9. Locate the outdoor mailbox closest to your home and get in the habit of walking to it to send off your bills or letters. Maybe it'll get you to write more letters—wonderful for your hands, even better for your friends and family.

10. If you have little children in your life—be they yours, grandchildren, nieces, nephews or even just neighbours—commit to the following per year: a trip to the ball game, a trip to the circus, a trip to the zoo, a trip to the aquarium and a trip to the kids' museum. Buy the tickets far in advance and exercise in advance so you're ready for a full day of fun.

11. Somehow, somehow, find a way to dance. Don't wait for a date or a wedding. Turn on the stereo and dance at home. Join a square-dance group or take ballroom lessons.

12. Come up with a personal "instant walk" trigger. For example, anytime you become drowsy, take a five-minute walk. Or, anytime you want a snack. Or, anytime you get angry, bored, melancholy or stressed. Walking isn't just an antidote for arthritis pain, it is a wonderful way to work out mental and emotional issues as well.

Shoulders help you maintain good posture and are critical for daily tasks ranging from carrying a bag of topsoil, picking a book off a shelf over your head or hoisting yourself out of a chair. Their wide range of motion makes strong shoulders essential to every upper-arm movement—forward, back, up, down or side to side. Their versatility also makes shoulders easy to injure, but you can protect them by making supporting muscles stronger. Here are 7 stretches and 10 exercises to do just that.

STRETCHES

Shoulder Roll

This stretch is helpful for people who hold muscle tension in the neck or upper back.

1. Stand up straight with feet hip-width apart and knees slightly bent. Relax your shoulders **a**. With arms down by your side, move your shoulders forward to stretch your shoulder blades, shrugging them toward your ears **b**. Move them backward so shoulder blades squeeze together and return to the starting position for a full backward circle. Do 6 repetitions.

2. From the starting position, repeat the exercise in the opposite direction, moving your shoulders back, up toward your ears in a shrugging motion, forward, then back down to the starting position, making a full forward circle.

TIP: Try to move in a smooth, continuous circular motion, making movements as large as is comfortable. Start with small circles and over time, try to make your circles bigger.

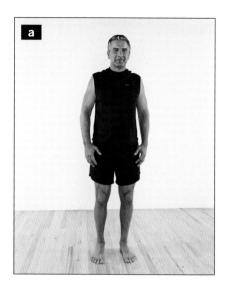

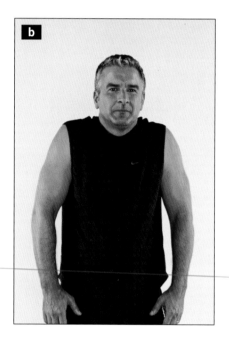

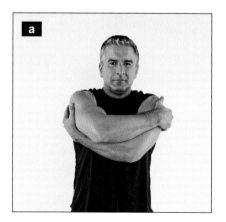

Self-Hug

1. Stand up straight with your feet hip-width apart and your knees slightly bent.

2. Wrap your arms around yourself, reaching each hand to grasp the opposite shoulder or the side of your torso to produce a stretch in the back of the shoulders. Hold.

Knuckle Rub

1. Stand up straight with feet hip-width apart and knees slightly bent, hands down by your side. Make a fist and, with knuckles facing forward, move your hands behind you and place your knuckles against your lower back.

2. Gently move your knuckles up your back until you feel a stretch in the front part of your shoulder and your upper arms 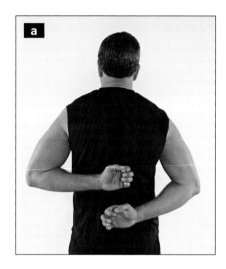. Hold.

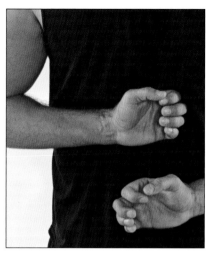

Wall Climb

This combination exercise stretches the shoulders in two directions and is especially good for people with a restricted range of shoulder motion. It also provides a workout for your fingers.

1. Stand up straight facing a wall from 18 inches (46 cm) away, with your feet hip-width apart, knees slightly bent and arms hanging down by your side.

2. Reach out with both arms and touch the wall at about waist level 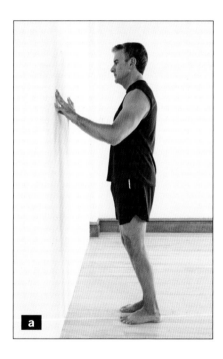. Use your fingers like spiders' legs to climb the wall until you feel a stretch at the back and sides of your shoulders. Hold. Slowly "climb" your fingers back down to waist level.

3. Turn so that your right hip is facing the wall from the same distance away 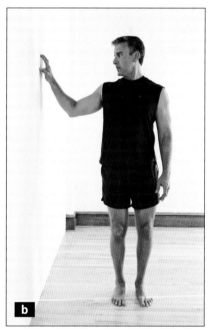. Reach out with your right hand and do the same spider-climb movement until you feel a stretch under your shoulder. Hold. Repeat on your left side.

Shoulder Twist

This exercise stretches the rotator cuff, a group of four muscles that stabilize the shoulder joint.

1. Stand straight with your feet hip-width apart and knees slightly bent, with arms hanging down by your side. Bend your elbows 90 degrees, keeping your upper arms next to your body so your forearms are parallel to the floor and pointed forward with thumbs pointing up (like shaking hands) **a**.

2. Keeping your thumbs up and elbows next to your body, move your hands away from each other until you feel a comfortable stretch in

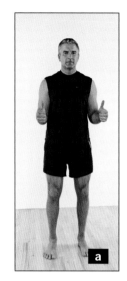
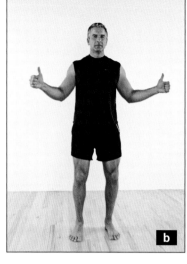
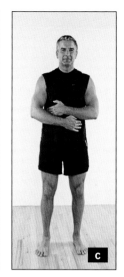

your shoulder **b**. Hold. Slowly bring your hands back toward you until the palms of your hands touch your body **c**. Hold.

TIP: On the return phase, to get palms to the front of your body, your hands will need to cross each other.

'Good Morning' Exercise

1. Stand straight with your feet hip-width apart and knees slightly bent, arms hanging down and hands on the front part of the opposite thigh.

2. Keeping your arms extended, lift your hands in a sideways and upward motion as high over your head as you can **a**. Hold for one second and return to the starting position. Do 6 repetitions.

TIP: Breathe in as you slowly lift your arms and exhale as you return, which helps you establish a rhythm and trains you to breathe more deeply.

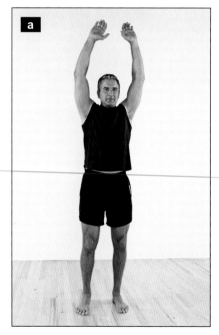

Scissors

This exercise stretches both the sides and backs of the shoulders.

1. Stand straight with your feet hip-width apart, arms by your side. With palms facing behind you, slowly swing your arms directly across the front of your body, with your right arm cutting in front of your left **a**.

2. Swing your arms back to the starting position, then cross them again, left arm cutting in front of the right. That is one repetition; do six.

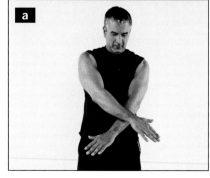

STRENGTH EXERCISES

LEVEL 1

Lying Lateral Raise

The flapping motion of this exercise provides a good all-around workout for muscles at the front, back and sides of the shoulders. Helpful for people who struggle to comb or wash their hair.

1. Lie on the floor or your bed with your arms by your side close to your body.

2. Slowly and smoothly move your extended arms out to the side so they are at shoulder level **a**. Slowly return to the starting position.

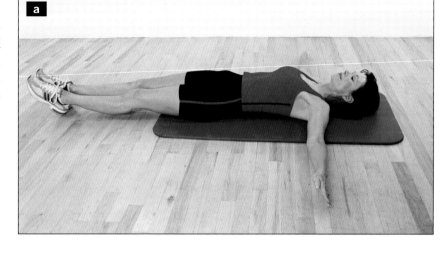

Lying Side Rotation

Here you work the shoulder's rotator cuff muscles as in the shoulder twist, but build strength by working against gravity.

1. Lie on the floor or a bed with legs extended and arms by your sides. Bend your elbows 90 degrees so that the tips of your fingers are facing the ceiling **a**.

2. Maintaining bent arms and keeping your elbows close to your body, slowly lower your hands to the sides as far as you comfortably can **b**. Slowly bring hands back to the starting position and beyond to touch the front of your body **c**.

NOTCH IT UP: To make this exercise more difficult, hold hand weights.

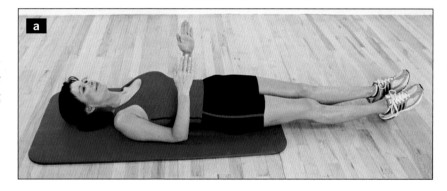

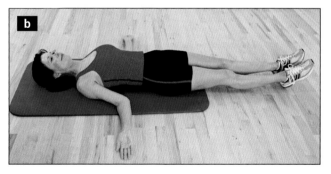

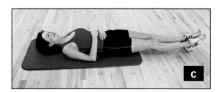

Shoulders >

everyday *secrets*

Be consistent. Always start exercises on the same side of the body. Consistency makes keeping track of repetitions easier, especially when one repetition is completed only after both sides of the body have performed the movement.

Get a beat on pain. To make exercise more comfortable, try applying heat to painful joints or taking pain-relieving medications before you start. Be careful not to push yourself too hard during the workout. Analgesics can mask "good" pain that would otherwise tell you to hold back.

Play with balloons. Challenge your grandchildren to a balloon-batting contest. The team that keeps it off the ground longest gets the prize, but everybody is a winner because this is a terrific exercise for building strength and range of motion in all the muscles of the upper extremities from shoulders and arms to wrists and fingers.

continued on page 84

Modified Around the World

This exercise helps to build mobility, strength and endurance for short over-the-head activities such as washing your hair.

1. Stand straight with your feet hip-width apart and knees slightly bent, arms hanging down and palms facing your thighs **a**. Slowly raise your extended arms out to the side until your hands reach the level of your shoulders **b**.

2. Keeping your arms at shoulder level, move your hands to the front and touch your thumbs together **c**. Slowly lower your arms in front of you until your palms touch the front of your thighs.

3. Do the entire exercise in reverse, raising hands to the front, moving them to the sides and lowering them back to the starting position to complete one repetition.

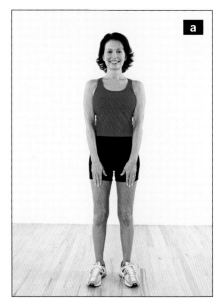

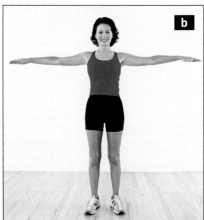

AT THE *Fitness Centre*

If you have access to good-quality exercise machines, here's what to use for your shoulders:

OVERHEAD PRESS
This exercise works like an overhead press using dumbbells, but guides your movement as you raise your arms against resistance.

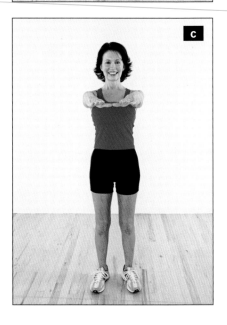

LEVEL 2

Upright Row

Some people have trouble bending their elbows enough to do this exercise completely at first, but regular practice helps build range of motion not only in your shoulders, but your elbows as well.

1. Stand straight with your feet hip-width apart and knees slightly bent, arms hanging down and hands resting on the front of your thighs.

2. Keeping your hands close to your body, slowly bring your hands up your front so that your elbows move out to the side until they reach about the level of your shoulders, with your hands at the level of your chest 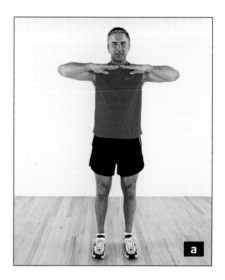. Hold for one second, then slowly lower your hands back to the starting position.

TIP: If it's difficult to raise your arms, just bring them to a level that feels comfortable.

NOTCH IT UP: To provide an extra challenge to muscles, hold a bit longer at the top of the lift. To significantly add resistance, hold hand weights.

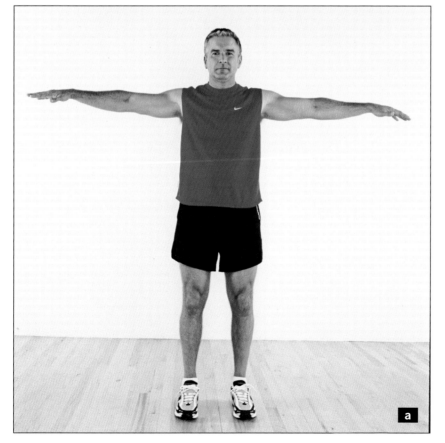

Standing Lateral Raise

This is the same basic movement as the lying lateral raises in level 1, but works more of the front, back and sides of the shoulders because you're working against gravity.

1. Stand straight with your feet hip-width apart and knees slightly bent, arms hanging down by your side, palms facing your body.

2. Keeping your arms extended, smoothly raise your hands out to the side until they reach the level of your shoulders 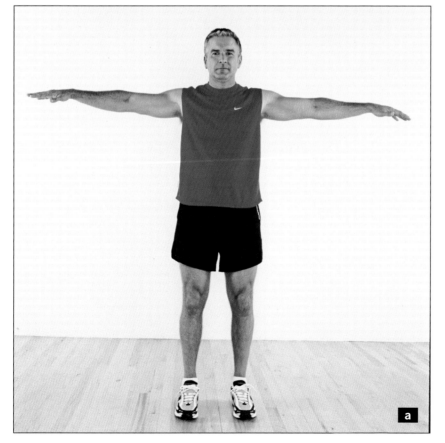. Slowly lower your hands to the starting position.

Front Raise

Varying the direction of the lift in this exercise concentrates resistance on the muscles at the front of your shoulders.

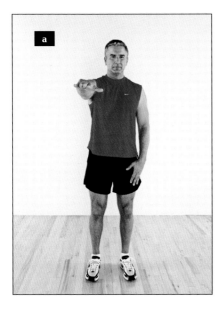

1. Stand straight with your feet hip-width apart and knees slightly bent, arms hanging down at the front of your thighs. Keeping your arms extended, slowly raise your right hand straight in front of you until it reaches the level of your shoulders **a**.

2. Slowly return to the starting position and repeat with the other arm to complete one repetition.

Around the World

This exercise works muscles surrounding the shoulder and helps develop coordinated movement. Similar to the modified around-the-world exercise in level 1, it requires you to lift your arms higher and extends your range of motion.

1. Stand straight with your feet hip-width apart and knees slightly bent, arms hanging down by your side and palms facing your thighs. Slowly raise your extended arms out to the side **a** until they go up over your head, turning your palms forward as you raise them so that your thumbs touch over your head **b**.

2. Slowly lower your extended arms in front of you until your palms touch the front of your thighs **c**. Reverse the move, raising your arms in front of you over your head, separating your hands and lowering your arms to the starting position to complete one repetition.

TIP: Make your movements smooth and fluid, not jerky, taking about three seconds to raise arms above your head, another three seconds to lower them to the front.

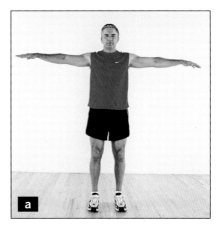

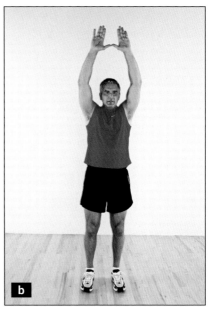

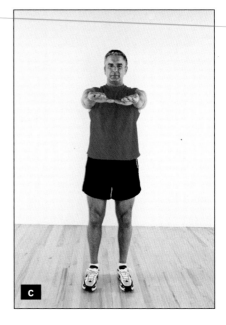

LEVEL 3

Weighted Lateral Raise

In a good example of how you can use the same basic exercise at three different levels of intensity, this move duplicates lateral raises in levels 1 and 2, but adds resistance with weights.

1. Stand straight with your feet hip-width apart and knees slightly bent, arms hanging down by your sides and a hand weight in each hand, palms facing your body.

2. Keeping your arms extended, slowly raise the weights out to the side until they reach the level of your shoulders **a**. Slowly lower the weights to the starting position.

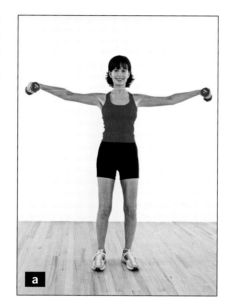

Weighted Front Raise

Again, the movement is the same as front raises in level 2, but weights add resistance and difficulty.

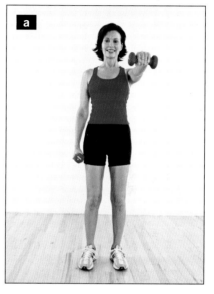

1. Stand straight with your feet hip-width apart and knees slightly bent. Grasp a hand weight in each hand, palms facing your body, arms hanging down at the front of your thighs. Keeping your arms extended, slowly raise the weight in your right hand straight in front of you until it reaches the level of your shoulders **a**.

2. Slowly return to the starting position and repeat with the left arm to complete one repetition.

Overhead Dumbbell Press

Your shoulders get an excellent workout in this classic exercise—and so do the muscles of your upper back and the back of your arms.

1. Sit on a straight-backed chair or an exercise bench holding a hand weight in each hand. Keeping your elbows close to your body, bring the weights up to your shoulders **a**. This is your starting position.

2. Take a breath and slowly exhale as you push the weights over your head, turning your hands so your palms face forward. Lift your arms as far as you comfortably can, but don't lock your elbows **b**. Slowly lower the weights to the starting position, turning your hands palms-inward as they come down.

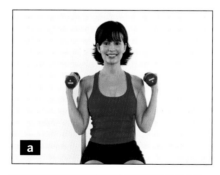

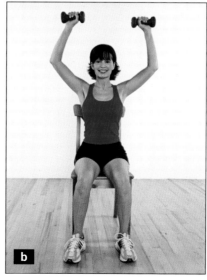

TIP: To avoid straining your joints, don't lock your elbows, but consistently keep your arms slightly bent through the entire exercise.

STRETCHES

Seated Torso Twist

1. Sit in a straight-backed chair, preferably one with arms, with feet flat on the floor and legs bent 90 degrees **a**.

2. Turn your upper body at the waist to the right so that you're looking over your right shoulder **b**. Relax and hold, breathing normally. Come back to the starting position and repeat on the other side.

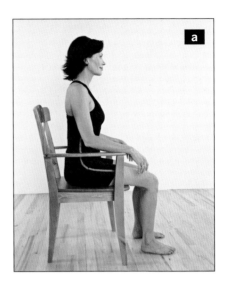

At first glance, having strong abs seems more important for looking good on the beach than beating arthritis. But these large muscles are critical for support of the torso and making them stronger contributes to improved posture—an important goal of physical activity for people with arthritis. Proper posture decreases stress throughout the body's joints, including those of the neck, spine, hips, knees and ankles. When your muscles and bones are in proper alignment, joints work more efficiently and you get better support from surrounding muscles, ligaments and tendons.

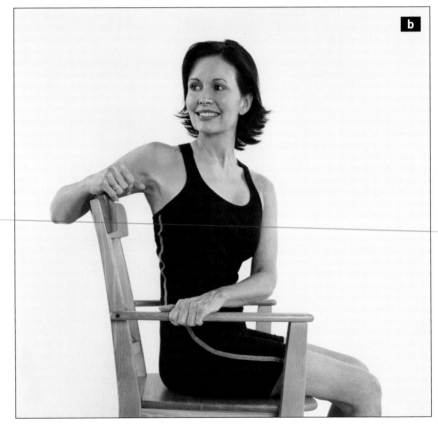

TIPS:
• To get an even better stretch, grab the arm of the chair to pull your body comfortably around using the hand on the side toward which you're twisting.

• If you're especially tight, do a second twist on each side after you finish your first complete set.

Ball Stretch

For this exercise, you'll need a fitness ball (scaled to your size) to provide a cushioned arch to your back that stretches the latticework of muscles throughout your abdomen.

1. Lie on your back with the ball positioned under your upper back, your hips lowered toward the floor and your knees bent about 90 degrees **a**.

2. Slowly straighten your knees so that you roll on your back along the ball, keeping your feet on the floor and your hands over your stomach—or wherever they feel most comfortable—until you feel a stretch in your abdominal area **b**.

TIPS:
• If you feel you need greater stability, place your feet wider than shoulder-width apart.

• As you become more confident using the ball, try putting your arms over your head, which enhances the stretch and challenges your balance, providing a mild workout for leg muscles.

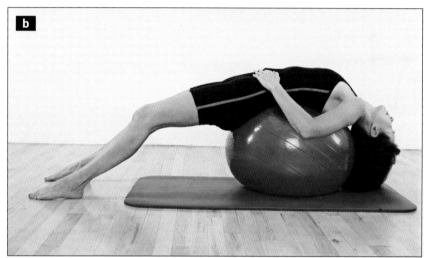

Lying Total Body Stretch

1. Lie on your back with your legs extended and feet together or about hip-width apart.

2. Extend your arms straight over your head and stretch your legs and toes, making your entire body as long as comfortably possible **a**. Hold.

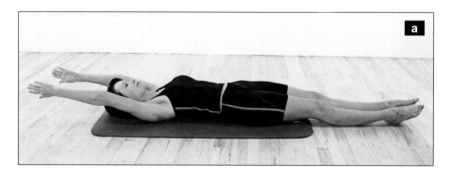

TIP: Take a deep breath before you begin the stretch and exhale as you extend your hands and feet, then breathe normally as you hold, which enhances the stretch. Don't hold your breath, which prevents the abdominal muscles from relaxing.

STRENGTH EXERCISES

LEVEL 1

Modified Abdominal Curl

The curl is a fundamental part of any well-rounded routine, but the hand position on this version creates less resistance than in a standard curl.

1. Lie on your back with feet flat on the floor, knees bent and your arms at your sides **a**.

2. Raising your head, use your abdominal muscles to pull your shoulders off the floor so you can look at the top of your knees **b**. Keep enough space to fit a baseball between your chin and chest as you come up and slide your hands forward along the floor as you move your shoulders off the floor.

3. Slowly lower your shoulders back to the floor.

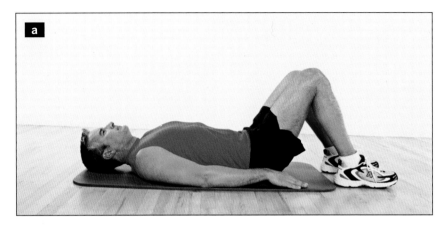

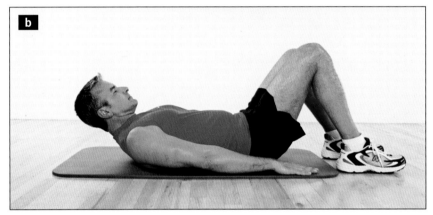

LEVEL 2

Basic Abdominal Curl

Start from the same position as in a modified curl (above), but with one difference: Put your hands across your chest, touching each hand to the opposite shoulder **a**. This provides more resistance for ab muscles to overcome **b**.

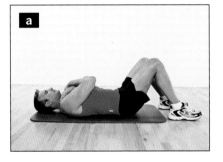

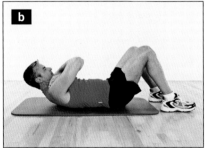

Basic Bicycle

This exercise is a favourite strength and endurance builder for athletes from diverse sports such as football, hockey, boxing, gymnastics, figure skating and martial arts—yet it's easy to modify so that even people with chronic musculoskeletal problems can perform it.

1. Lie flat on your back with your legs straight and your hands behind or lightly touching your ears.

2. Lift your head off the floor and bring your left knee toward your head, stopping when your knee is about waist level and your thigh is perpendicular to the floor. At the same time, bring your right elbow toward the elevated knee so that your torso twists slightly and

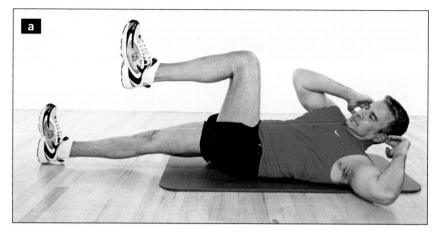

your elbow and knee are as close as possible over your abdomen **a**.

3. Slowly return to the starting position. Rest for one second and repeat with the opposite limbs.

TIP: This exercise should take about 5 seconds, with 2 seconds to bring knee and elbow close and 3 seconds to return. As you become stronger, reduce the resting time for a more difficult workout. All motions should be smooth and controlled, which keeps resistance on muscles longer and improves strength and tone more quickly.

Flutter Kick

This exercise helps build abdominal strength, but also enhances coordination if you swim.

1. Lie on your back, propped on your elbows, with your feet straight out in front of you, toes pointed toward the ceiling **a**.

2. Lift your right heel 4 to 6 inches off the ground **b**. Bring it back to the floor, then lift and return the left leg in the same way to complete one repetition. Continue this kicking motion until you finish a set.

TIP: Though this move resembles swimming, don't kick fast like you're in the water, but keep movements slow and controlled, taking one second to lift and one second to return.

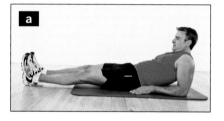

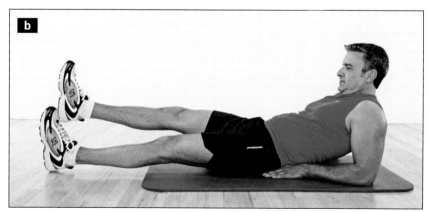

Abdomen >

everyday
secrets

Use the stairs. The familiar advice to take stairs instead of an elevator seems like a great way to build exercise into your day—if you don't work on the 14th floor. But don't think "all or nothing." You can walk up to the second floor, catch the elevator there and ride the rest of the way. As you get stronger, take more flights and ride less.

Try two for one. Taking stairs two at a time doubles the exercise—you get the benefits of stair-climbing plus lunging. (And you may even beat the elevator.)

Walk, don't slouch. You can enhance the benefits of walking by practising good posture as you stride. Hold your body so that shoulders and hips are aligned without arching your back. Keep your elbows close to your body. Let arms swing freely forward and back in a straight line.

continued on page 90

LEVEL 3

Advanced Abdominal Curl

Lift your head and shoulders off the floor just as you do with modified and basic curls, but in this version, touch your hands lightly behind your ears, which adds even greater resistance **a** .

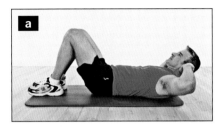

TIP: Don't hold your head in your hands to do curls. That tends to make you pull your head up with your hands, which puts pressure on the back of your upper spine. Instead, touch your hands lightly behind your ears **b** .

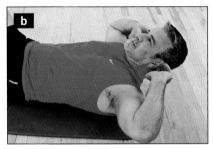

Advanced Flutter Kick

As with the flutter kick in level 2, you move your feet up and down as if swimming. In this exercise, however, you start with both feet 1 to 2 inches (2.5 to 5 cm) off the ground and keep them elevated through the entire exercise **a** . Take slightly less time to complete one kick, lifting in a half second and returning in a half second (or whatever speed feels most comfortable) **b** .

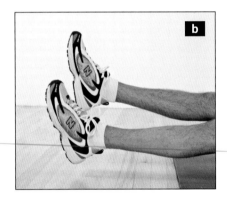

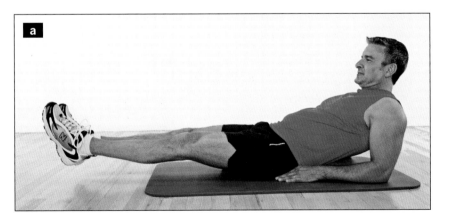

Advanced Bicycle

The movements with this exercise are the same as the basic bicycle in level 1. The difference:

With this advanced version, in the starting position, hold both your heels one to two inches off the floor and keep both feet elevated through the entire exercise. At the same time, hold your head and shoulders off the floor **a**. This constant resistance prevents rest between repetitions, making the advanced bicycle considerably more difficult than the basic version **b**.

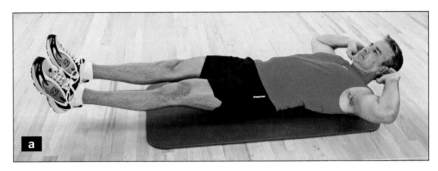

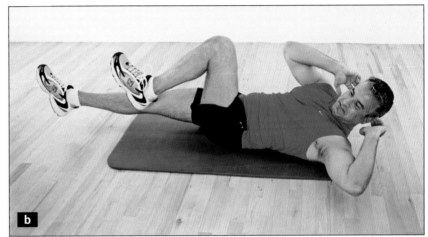

Ball Curl

Consider this exercise a how-low-can-you-go challenge—but use an exercise ball instead of a limbo bar.

1. Sit up straight on the ball, crossing each hand across your chest to touch the opposite shoulder. Place feet flat on the floor, with your knees bent at about 90 degrees **a**.

2. Slowly lean backward while keeping the ball from rolling **b**. Lean back as far as you can while still maintaining balance. Slowly return to the starting position for one repetition.

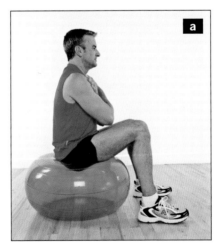

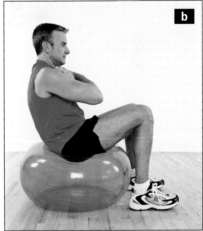

TIP: Don't worry about achieving a certain angle with your backward lean: The idea is to move as far as is comfortable—but if you consistently do the exercise, you'll make strides in both strength and balance that will allow you to lean back farther.

NOTCH IT UP: To make this exercise even more difficult, put your hands by your ears, which transfers weight to your upper body and increases resistance on your abdominal muscles.

Arthritis in the spine causes pain and stiffness, but can also lead to effects elsewhere in the body, such as weakness in the arms or legs. Getting up and walking is one of the most important ways to exercise the back, but you can also target the muscles that support the spine and help protect its joints. Even if you don't have arthritis in your spine, the torso-building exercises in this section can help prevent back pain—an exceedingly common condition—from making arthritis seem worse.

STRETCHES

Standing Posture Exercise

Your posture may suffer if arthritis has made you guard your movements by, for example, rounding your shoulders or leaning to one side. This exercise helps train your body to maintain proper alignment.

1. Stand with your back against a wall with your heels as close to the wall as possible.

2. Touch the wall with your shoulders and the back of your head **a**. Register how your body feels in this good-posture position. Hold for 15 to 30 seconds—but try to carry yourself in this position as much as possible throughout your day.

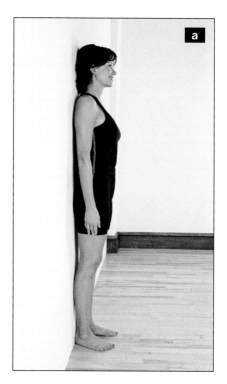

Low Back Knees to Chest

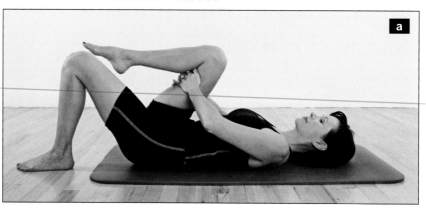

Though similar to the knees-to-chest exercise in the knees and hips section, this exercise keeps one foot flat on the floor, which bypasses the hip flexor muscles and provides a better stretch for the lower back.

1. Lie on your back with your right leg fully extended and your left knee bent with the foot flat on the floor. Bring your right knee up to the level of your waist, keeping your left foot planted.

2. Put your hands in the crook of your leg behind your right thigh and gently pull your knee toward your right shoulder **a**. Stop when you feel a slight stretch. Hold and gently return to the starting position. Repeat on the other side.

Pelvic Twist

1. Lie on your back with your knees bent, feet flat on the floor and arms extended straight out to your sides **a**.

2. Gently lower both knees to your right side until you feel a slight stretch in your left lower back and hip area **b**. Hold and return to the starting position. Repeat on the other side.

TIP: To get the most from this stretch, keep both shoulders on the floor.

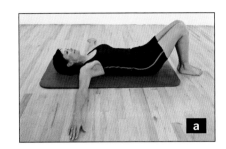

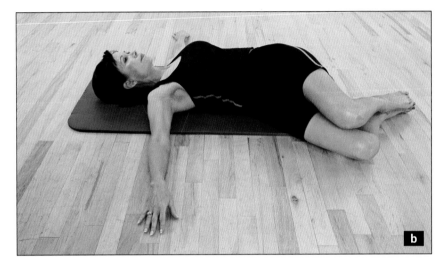

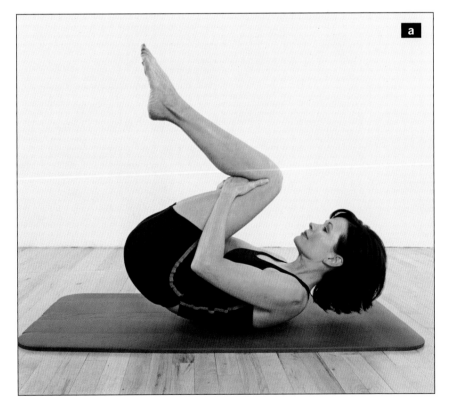

Rocking Chair

The rocking motion of this stretch helps develop muscle control and, by contracting the stomach muscles, automatically causes the nervous system to relax back muscles, allowing a better stretch.

1. Lie on your back with knees bent and feet flat on the floor. Reach up and put your hands behind your knees.

2. Pull both knees toward your shoulders. When you feel a slight stretch in your lower back and buttocks, gently rock back and forth on your rounded back **a**.

TIP: This exercise is most comfortable when done on a rug, exercise mat or bed.

Cat Stretch

This is a classic back stretch, often used in yoga routines.

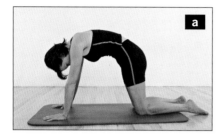

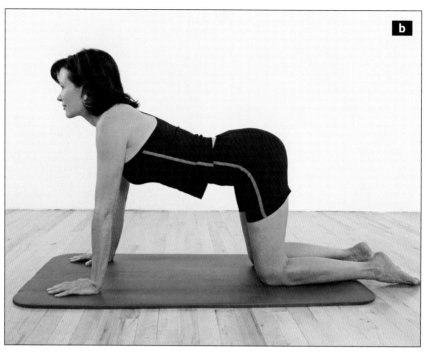

1. Get on your hands and knees. Tuck your chin toward your chest and tighten your stomach muscles to arch your back **a**. Hold.

2. Relax, raising your head so you're looking straight ahead while pushing your stomach toward the floor **b**. Hold.

Cross-Legged Seated Stretch

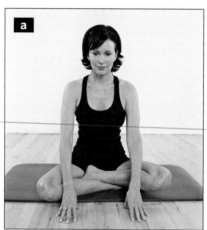

1. Sit on the floor with your legs crossed and hands in front of you **a**. Lean forward gently with your head down, rounding your back and "walking" your fingers forward until you feel a stretch in your lower and middle back **b**. Hold.

2. Walk your hands back to your legs and return to the starting position.

TIP: For a balanced stretch to both sides of the back, do this exercise twice, switching the leg that is crossed over the top.

>STRETCHES

Seated Body Hang

If you feel light-headed when you lean over, skip this stretch.

1. Sit in a straight-backed chair (with or without arms), with your feet flat on the floor and your hands on your knees **a**.

2. Gently lean forward, moving your hands toward the floor between your feet until you feel a stretch in your middle and lower back **b**. Hold.

TIP: To return to the starting position if you have back pain, put your hands or forearms on your knees and push yourself up.

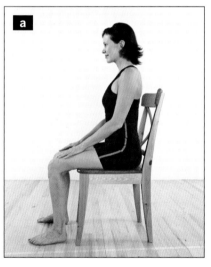

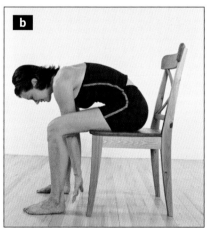

Side Bend and Twist

In the second part of this move, raising your hands helps keep your head in proper alignment with your upper body.

1. Stand straight with your feet about hip-width apart, arms at your sides.

2. Gently lean to the right, sliding your hand down the side of your thigh toward your knee until you feel a slight stretch on the left side of your waist **a**. Hold. Return to the starting position and repeat on the other side.

3. Return to the starting position and bend your elbows at about 90 degrees so that your hands are in front of you. Rotate your upper body so that your hands move to the right side while keeping your hips pointed straight ahead until you feel a stretch in your left lower back **b**. Hold.

4. Slowly return to the starting position and repeat on the other side.

TIP: If you feel unbalanced during the side bend, place your feet farther apart for greater stability or try a similar move from a sitting position.

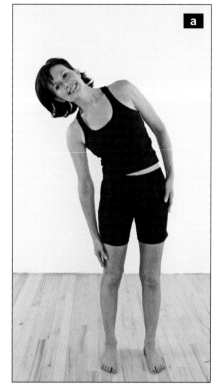

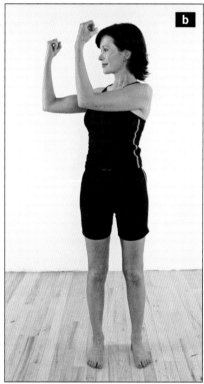

Back and Spine >

continued on page 97

everyday *secrets*

Try intervals. If walking seems too tame, but running is too hard on your joints, try a technique called interval training, in which you crank up the pace periodically— but only for short spurts. Example: Walk at your normal pace for 5 minutes, then walk much faster for 30 seconds—then slow back down to your usual stride for another 5 minutes and repeat. This sequence boosts intensity, but poses minimal risk of injury.

Grip the bike right. Grip the handlebars firmly enough to control the bike, but loosely enough to keep hand and arm muscles from being unnecessarily tense. Keep your elbows slightly bent.

Add music to your motion. Add a portable CD player to your fitness gear and use it on your walks. Music has been shown to have a measurable impact on performance. In one Ohio State University study, walking-program participants who listened to music on the road covered 21 percent more miles after eight weeks than walkers who didn't tread to tunes.

STRENGTH EXERCISES

LEVEL 1

Lying Alternating Arm Raise

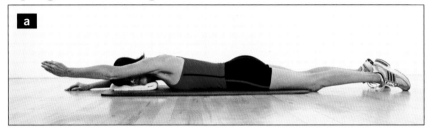

This exercise focuses on the muscles of the neck, upper back and shoulder blade area.

1. Lie on your stomach with your legs extended, your head straight down on a pillow or folded towel or turned to the side, whichever is more comfortable and your arms extended directly in front of you.

2. Smoothly raise your left arm as far as comfortably possible [a]. Hold one second and lower. Repeat with the other arm to complete one repetition.

Lower-Body Extension

This exercise is not only excellent for the hips (you'll find it in that section as well), but also works the muscles of the lower back.

1. Get down on your hands and knees on the floor, a rug or an exercise mat.

2. Extend your left leg out behind you, keeping your foot about one inch off the floor as you straighten your knee [a]. Return to the starting position and repeat with the other leg to complete one repetition.

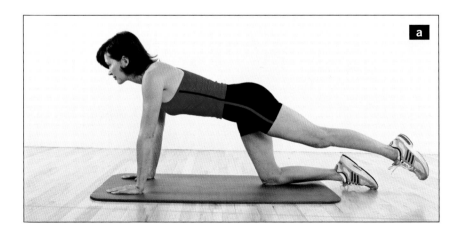

LEVEL 2

Superman

This exercise hits muscles through-out the spine from the base of your head to the buttocks, all of which add stability to your spine.

1. Lie on your stomach with your arms extended directly in front of you, your legs straight out behind you and your eyes looking at your hands **a** .

2. Holding your chin off the floor, gently lift both arms and both feet about 1 inch (2.5 cm), hold one second and lower to the floor for one repetition **b** .

TIP: If you feel discomfort in the back of your neck, keep your eyes facing the floor and rest your head on a pillow instead of lifting your chin off the floor.

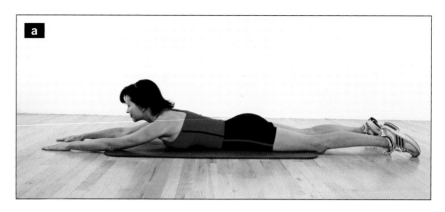

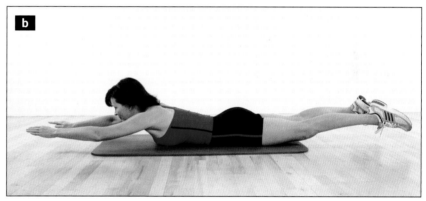

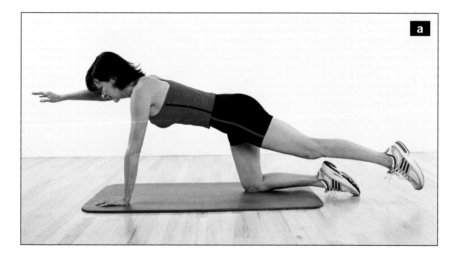

Bird Dog

As with the lower-body extension, this exercise works muscles in both the back and hips, so it's an excel-lent choice for either area (see also Knees and Hips, page 66).

1. Get down on your hands and knees on the floor, a rug or an exercise mat.

2. Extend your left leg out behind you, keeping your foot about 1 inch (2.5 cm) off the floor as you straighten your knee. At the same time you extend your left leg, reach out straight in front of you with your right arm **a** .

3. Return to the starting position and repeat with the other leg and arm to complete one repetition.

Back and Spine >

Bent Single Arm Row

This exercise is best done on an exercise bench, but can also be performed using a sturdy armless chair.

1. Stand by the front corner of an armless chair with your feet about hip-width apart, holding a hand weight in your right hand.

2. Bend over and place your left hand on the chair so that your back is parallel with the floor. Lower the weight so your right arm is straight **a**.

3. Lift the weight toward your chest, holding your elbow close to your body and moving it straight up toward the ceiling. Stop when the weight is just below chest level

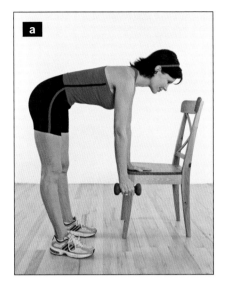

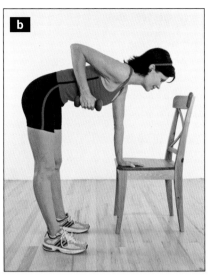

b. Hold for one second and slowly lower the weight to the straight-arm starting position. After completing a set, repeat with the other arm.

TIP: If you have pain or discomfort in the hand or wrist you lean on, instead rest your elbow and forearm on the back of the chair for support.

LEVEL 3

Dead Lift

If your function level is good and you perform the movement correctly, this exercise will strengthen your lower back and build better posture.

1. Stand with your feet about hip-width apart, knees slightly bent **a**.

2. Keeping knees slightly flexed, bend over at the waist and lower your hands straight down toward your feet, keeping your hands close to your legs at first, then moving them out to your toes **b**. Return to the standing position for one repetition.

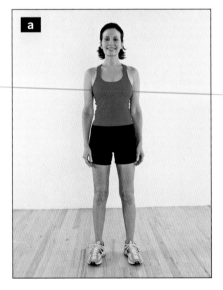

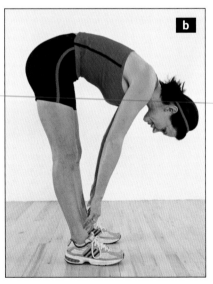

TIPS:
• Avoid this exercise if you have back problems or lower back pain.

• If you lack flexibility in hamstrings and hips, start by bending so hands go only to knee. Don't lock your knees.

NOTCH IT UP: You make this exercise more difficult—and more worthy of caution—by using hand weights. Attempt this only after you've developed strength and flexibility in your lower back by doing the exercise without weights.

Advanced Bird Dog

Building on the basic bird dog move in level 2, this more advanced exercise not only works the muscles of the hips, but also the back and shoulders.

1. Get down on your hands and knees on the floor, a rug or an exercise mat.

2. Extend your left leg out behind you, raising your foot so that your entire leg is parallel to the floor—a more strenuous position than in the basic bird dog. At the same time, reach out straight in front of you with your right arm **a**.

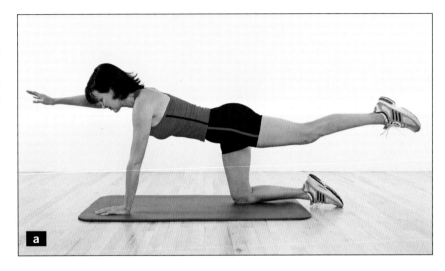

3. Return to the starting position and repeat with the other leg and arm to complete one repetition. Continue alternating legs and arms until you finish a set.

AT THE *Fitness Centre*

If you have access to good-quality exercise machines, here's what to use for your back and spine:

SEATED ROW MACHINE
For best results, if you have a choice of handle grips, select one in which the handles are vertical; if there are multiple grip positions, choose the innermost one.

PULL-DOWN MACHINE
You may see other exercisers pulling the bar behind their heads, but it's best to avoid such a move, which puts excess stress on the shoulder joint. Do the exercise in a slow and controlled manner, keeping your back straight so you don't use any momentum to pull the bar down. To make this exercise more difficult, place your hands closer to the ends of the bar. For another variation, rotate your palms to face inward (as if doing a chin-up) and position your hands 2 to 3 inches (5 to 7 cm) apart, which works muscles lower down the sides of your back.

Chest muscles play a vital role in stabilizing the multidirectional shoulder joints, which are essential to a wide variety of every-day tasks, such as carrying heavy loads and opening doors. Building strong chest muscles also helps improve posture, taking pressure off the spine. What's more, many exercises for chest muscles also work the hands and arms, conditioning muscles from all of these areas to work together.

STRETCHES

Seated Chest Stretch

This stretch for the upper chest and front shoulders can be done from either a standing or sitting position.

1. Place your hands at the back of your head with fingers interlocked **a**.

2. Gently move your elbows backward or behind you until you feel a stretch at the front of your shoulders and the top of your chest **b**.

TIP: If you find you're especially stiff in this area, assume the starting position in a straight-backed chair and have a partner assist by gently pulling your elbows back from behind the chair. As soon as you feel a slight stretch in your chest, tell your partner to stop pulling. Or do the stretch lying on your back with knees bent and both feet flat on the floor.

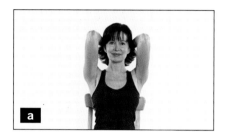

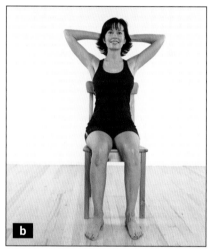

Lying Total Body Stretch

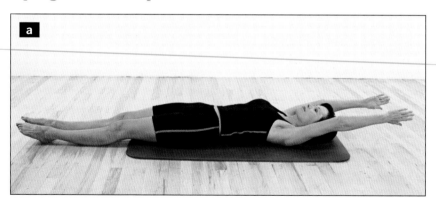

By putting your hands over your head, this stretch (a double–duty move also described in the abdominal section, page 81) lengthens chest muscles in a different direction than the other stretches.

1. Lie on your back on a bed or a mat with your legs extended and feet together or comfortably apart at about hip width.

2. Extend your arms straight over your head and stretch your legs and toes, making your entire body as long as comfortably possible **a**. Hold.

Wall Stretch

1. Start by standing with your right side next to a wall, then take one regular-size step forward with your left foot. Place your right forearm vertically against the wall, with your elbow bent at 90 degrees so that your upper arm is parallel to the floor and your hand is pointing toward the ceiling.

2. Keeping your back heel flat on the floor, slowly bend your front knee so that your body moves forward and you feel a stretch in your chest and upper arm **a**. Hold and repeat on the other side.

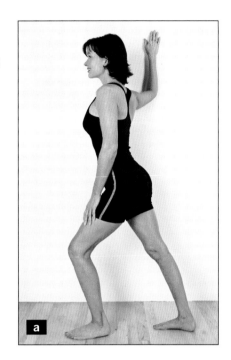

STRENGTH EXERCISES

LEVEL 1

Wall Push-Up

1. From a standing position about 12 to 18 inches (30 to 46 cm) from a wall, put your hands on the wall about shoulder-width apart at chest level, with palms flat and fingers pointed toward the ceiling **a**.

2. Slowly lower your chin toward the wall **b**. Smoothly push back from the wall to the starting position.

TIP: As you lower yourself to the wall, keep elbows out to the side. That works the chest muscles better than keeping elbows close to the body, which shifts the load more to the triceps muscles of the arms. If you feel pain in your hands or wrist, try placing hands farther apart or closer together on the wall, which may prove more comfortable. If not, you may want to choose another exercise.

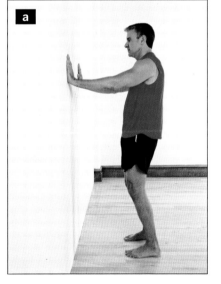

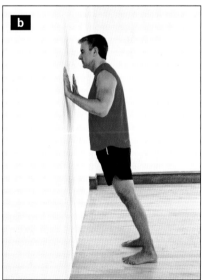

Chest >

Chest Fly

This is a weightlifting move without the weight. But if you're not already strength training, this exercise can make you stronger without causing soreness from working against too much resistance.

1. Lie on the floor with knees bent and feet flat. Extend your hands toward the ceiling with your arms slightly bent, palms facing each other **a**.

2. Slowly inhale as you lower your extended arms until your hands are just above the floor **b**. Hold for one second and, exhaling, raise your extended arms and bring your hands together at the starting position.

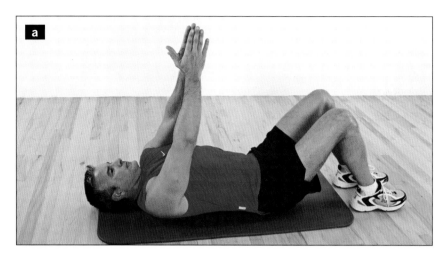

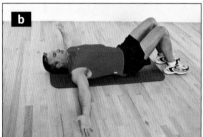

TIP: Keep your elbows slightly bent through the entire movement, not changing the angle, which would alter the amount of resistance on the muscles of the chest. This exercise can also be done lying on a bed.

LEVEL 3

Weighted Chest Fly

This exercise follows the same basic motion as the chest fly in level 1, but adds hand weights for greater resistance. While this is best done on an exercise bench, a floor mat will do.

1. Place your hand weights in a convenient location on either side of a floor mat, then lie down on your back with knees bent and feet flat to the floor, shoulder-width apart. Carefully grab your hand weights and press them toward the ceiling, holding them with palms facing each other **a**. This is your starting position.

2. Maintaining a slight bend in your elbow, inhale as you smoothly lower the weights to your sides until your upper arm is nearly parallel to the

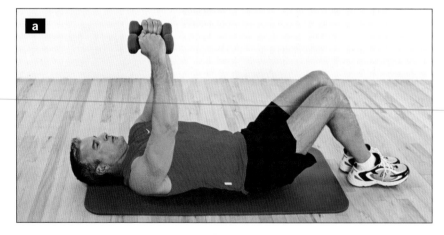

floor **b**. Try not to put the weights on the floor, but rather hold them a few inches (7 or 8 cm) above. Exhale as you pull your hands back up toward the starting position.

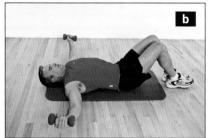

TIP: Keep your lifting movement smooth and controlled to cut momentum and prevent the weights from knocking against each other at the top of the lift.

LEVEL 3

Ball Push-Up

This exercise is even more challenging than a traditional push-up (which you could use as a level 2 exercise) because you need to draw on stabilizing muscles to keep the ball from rolling from side to side.

1. Put the fitness ball against a wall and place your hands on the top of the ball about shoulder-width apart, with your arms straight, your legs extended and your feet about hip-width apart.

2. Inhaling, slowly lower yourself until your chest touches the ball **a**. Exhaling, push your body away from the ball to the starting position.

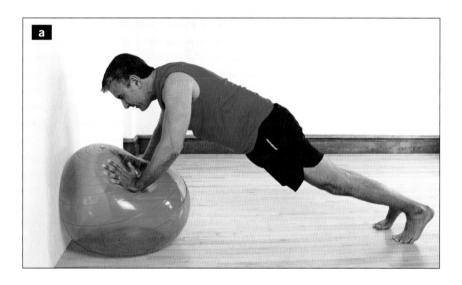

AT THE *Fitness Centre*

If you have access to good-quality exercise machines, here's what to use for your chest:

CHEST PRESS MACHINE
Keep your elbows aligned with your hands through the entire exercise to avoid putting excessive pressure on the hand joints. When grabbing hold, make sure the bar is pressing on the pad of your palm. If the bar isn't padded and you find it uncomfortable, try placing a sponge or towel in your hand as you grip the bar for added cushioning—but be careful this doesn't compromise your grip. Doing one set places this exercise at level 2; adding sets as you get stronger notches it up to level 3.

everyday *secrets*

Break it up. Sitting still—hunched over a desk or a computer station, for example—can cause tension and strain that makes muscles and joints more painful. To avoid this discomfort, take a short break at least every 10 minutes or so (set a timer if you're really concentrating). Stand up and walk around for a minute; it relieves tension (especially in the back) and mildly exercises stiff muscles and joints.

Make breaks automatic. While working at your desk, stash items that you use occasionally (but not constantly) beyond your reach. That way, you'll be forced to get up every now and then—in effect, taking a break and mildly exercising without feeling like you've stopped working.

Play ball. Just because it's fitness equipment doesn't mean you can't have fun with an exercise ball. Example: Making a lunge to bounce a ball against a wall with your hands provides a workout for wrist, hands, shoulders, chest, back, hips and knees.

continued on page 100

Your neck muscles are probably fairly strong already because they're accustomed to handling an ample amount of resistance: the weight of your head. But that's not all neck muscles do. They also help maintain proper posture, which relieves stress on the overall structure of the neck and spine and are critical for daily functions such as looking over your shoulder when backing out of a parking space. Daily demands go a long way toward keeping neck muscles in shape. Yet in some cases, constant muscular tension in the neck can contribute to headaches and back pain, especially if arthritis makes you limit your head movement. Your goal, then, isn't to progressively build strength, but to improve flexibility, tone and endurance. That's why the exercises in this section can be done at all three function levels. To progress, simply add repetitions as you become stronger and more comfortable.

STRETCHES

Neck Side Bend

1. Sit up straight in a chair with your eyes looking directly ahead **a**.

2. Slowly lower your right ear toward your right shoulder, stopping when you feel a slight stretch in the muscles on the left side of your neck **b**. Hold. Return to the starting position and repeat on the other side.

TIP: The weight of your head is sufficient to produce a good stretch for functional (but not excessive) range of motion—so there's no need to pull the side of your head down with your hand. You can do a similar stretch for muscles at the back of your neck by slowly letting your head dip forward. However, avoid stretching your neck by leaning your head back: This position can interfere with blood supply to the brain and may cause faintness.

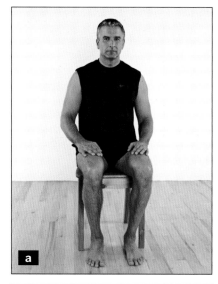

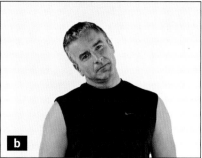

Neck Turn

You can do this exercise anytime, anywhere, while sitting or standing. But if your neck is sensitive or in pain, do this exercise lying down to lessen the pressure.

1. Sit or stand up straight with your eyes looking directly ahead.

2. Slowly and smoothly move your head to the right side until you feel a slight stretch in the muscles on the opposite side of your neck **a**. Relax and hold. Slowly return to the starting position and repeat on the other side.

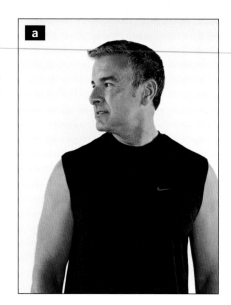

Posture Stretch

You might think this doesn't qualify as a stretching exercise—there's virtually no physical effort involved. Still, this visualizing exercise has excellent posture-building benefits.

1. While standing with feet about hip-width apart, imagine that there's a string attached to the top of your head pulling you up and making you an inch taller and adjust your body accordingly **a**. This will help you understand what it feels like to sit up straight, eliminate rounding of the shoulders and

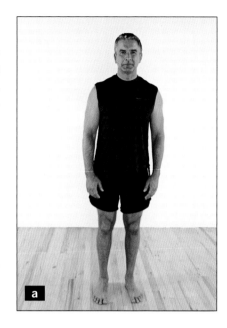

align your head and neck. Practising this mind/body exercise continuously will automatically improve your posture and make your entire body fall into better alignment, easing muscle tension and helping to relieve pain.

TIP: Don't push up with your toes when doing this exercise standing: The goal is to *feel* like you're being pulled up an inch; you don't actually need to be taller. If you have trouble standing straight or have pain in the hips or knees, perform this exercise sitting in a chair.

STRENGTH EXERCISES

'Yes' Exercise

This isometric exercise can be done almost anywhere.

1. Sit in a chair with your back against the chair and your neck slightly bent forward as if you're nodding yes **a**.

2. Press your head forward while applying gentle resistance to your forehead with either a pillow or your palms **b**. Hold as follows, according to your function level:

• 3 seconds for level 1
• 6 seconds for level 2
• 10 seconds for level 3

Relax and repeat one more time.

3. Press your head backward while applying gentle resistance by placing both hands behind your head with fingers interlaced **c**.

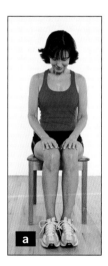
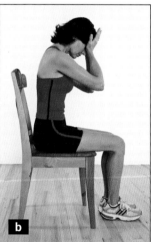
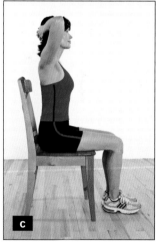

TIP: For a variation on the pressing-forward phase, get a similar effect using gravity by lying on your back and lifting your head an inch or two (2.5 to 5 cm) off the floor—as if you're doing an abdominal curl, but without raising your shoulders off the floor. The pressing-back phase of this exercise looks relaxing, but it shouldn't be. Actively push your head back against your hands.

everyday *secrets*

Use good phone technique. One of the most common causes of tension in the cervical spine is sloppy use of the telephone. It's not enough to stop cradling the handset between your ear and shoulder. You should also avoid holding it on just one side of your head— switch hands (and ears) regularly during a conversation. If you have a cell phone, use the hands-free earpiece/microphone that's included with it. Otherwise, pick up one at an electronics store.

Create a pain-free desk. Rearrange your desk to eliminate sources of strain on muscles and joints. Keep the objects you use often in a semi-circle within arm's reach. When you grab something, bring it close to your body to use. Heavy objects such as reference books should be on your desk or a middle shelf nearby. Avoid reaching for objects over your head or behind you, especially if they're heavy. Stand up to get them.

continued on page 106

Resisted Side Press

Think of this as a side-to-side version of the "yes" exercise.

1. Sit up straight in a chair with your eyes focused forward and your head cocked slightly to the right.

2. Press your head toward your right shoulder while applying gentle resistance with the heel of your right hand against the side of your head above the ear **a**. Relax and repeat on the other side.

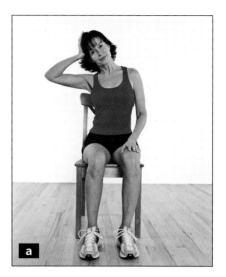

MASSAGES

Side Stroke

1. Place the fingers of your left hand on the right side of your neck just below your ear and stroke muscles in a downward motion toward your collarbone **a**.

2. Lift your fingers and return to the starting position. Do three strokes and repeat on the other side.

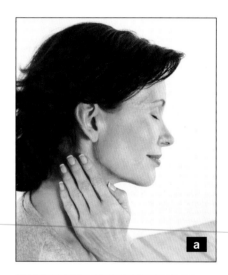

Vertebrae Press

1. Place your left hand on the back of your neck with fingers positioned on the right side of the neck bones just below the hairline.

2. Press with your fingers as you move your hand along the cervical spine from the base of your head to your shoulder **a**. Do this three times and repeat on the other side.

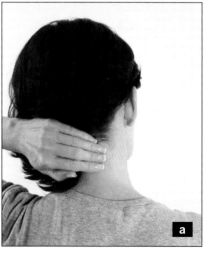

9 Ways to Prevent Stressed Muscles

For many people, the stresses of life—be they mental or physical—show up quickly in the neck muscles. Stretches and exercises can relieve a neck ache, but here are nine ways to avoid having your body tense up in the first place. And all are particularly good for arthritis as well!

1. Be like a cat and stretch often—and luxuriously. Your body wants to stretch and often does so unconsciously. Stretching loosens the muscles, helps your blood flow, relieves your bones and joints and refreshes your spirit. For a person with arthritis, stretching is as healthy a habit as you can develop. It can be a formal, multi-step routine or it can be just standing up and exalting the sky.

2. Find more reasons to laugh. The obvious reason is that humour relieves the tensions of everyday life. But not so obvious are the physiological effects of a good laugh. Feel-good brain chemicals called endorphins are released when you laugh that ease pain and improve attitude. Plus, laughter stimulates the heart, lungs, muscles and immune system.

3. Chop your to-do list in half. We know we're not going to get everything done that we want to in a day. And yet so many of us wake up with a set of expectations for the day that are grand beyond reason. Be fair to yourself: Make your task list reasonable and achieve it. There's no better way to reduce physical and emotional stress than regularly feeling like a success.

4. Glory in hot water. The water soothes and supports the joints. The heat brings blood to your joints, muscles and skin, flushing you with nutrients and relief. And the calmness of a soak in a tub or Jacuzzi makes life just seem better. Ask your doctor first if a Jacuzzi habit is healthy for you—the heat can alter your circulation.

5. Invest in your bed (and your bedding). There are pillows and then there are pillows. Same for mattresses, mattress pads, sheets and comforters. A bed that is firm but luxurious, that makes you say "ahhhh" when you lie down, that gives you the comfort you need for a great night's sleep, is a wonderful investment for your health and your joints.

6. Create a midday ritual. Perhaps it's a cup of tea, a walk, a stretch, a music break or just a phone call. Whatever it is, take 5 to 15 minutes each afternoon for a personal break. Getting out of the intensity of everyday life for a short while is beneficial, both physically and emotionally. And by making it a constant ritual, you relax yourself merely by the knowledge that it is soon arriving.

7. Trust us: A good massage is one of life's greatest pleasures. Every month or so, skip the weekend trip to the hair salon and spend the money instead on a massage. The muscle and joint relief will be substantial.

8. Live your life in ebbs and flows. In exploring the optimal workouts for athletes, researchers are beginning to believe that the best training method is to exert for a short period and then rest, rather than doing prolonged periods of exertion. It's a theory that is applicable to all of us, particularly those with arthritis. Walk a few minutes; then relax a while. Clean for 15 minutes; then take a break. This way, you don't overtax muscles and you give all the parts of your body a chance to recover before exerting again.

9. Let it be. If you are a human being, then certain truths are inevitable: The government is wrong; half your relatives are crazy; there's never enough money; work is unfair; you're surrounded by crazy drivers. You have a choice: Let it get to you or don't let it get to you. Our recommendation: When a cause for anger dangles in front of you, don't take the bait. Life's too short to be angry all the time. And it's not fair to your body.

The muscles of the ankles and feet are small. You can give them a good workout using simple exercises with only small amounts of resistance. These exercises use body weight rather than special equipment. But the size of muscles isn't a measure of their importance: The muscles that support the ankle and foot joints are critical to your mobility in walking and climbing stairs. Body-weight exercises are ideal because they train the muscles in the ways you actually use them in daily life.

STRETCHES

Stair Calf Stretch

1. Stand on a stair with feet about hip-width apart, with your weight on the balls of your feet and your heels sticking over the edge of the stair **a**.

2. Slowly lower your heels until you feel a stretch in your calves and the backs of your ankles **b**. Hold and return to the starting position.

TIP: Hold on to the stair rail or wall to steady yourself and maintain control during the stretch. Because your entire body weight factors into this stretch, be careful not to drop your heels too far or too fast—and be sure to stretch both legs at once.

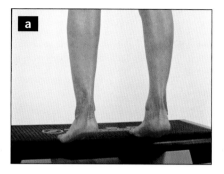

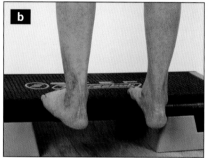

Ankle Circle

This is not a static stretch, but a range-of-motion exercise that promotes ankle mobility.

1. Sit in a chair with legs extended slightly so that heels rest on the floor about hip-width apart and toes point up at about a 45-degree angle.

2. Rotate from your ankles in a clockwise direction so that your toes trace circles in the air **a**. Do this 6 to 8 times.

3. Change direction, making counter-clockwise circles.

TIPS:
• If you're comfortable making small circles, expand your range of motion by pushing or pulling toes as far in each

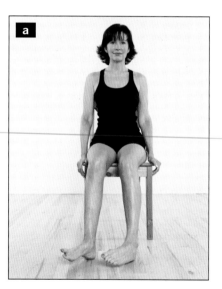

direction as you can. Your feet don't have to touch. For example, you could do this exercise with feet dangling as you sit on the edge of your bed.

• To add a simultaneous resistance exercise for your legs, elevate your feet while performing the ankle motion.

Runner's Calf Stretch

Always a popular way for runners to limber up their calves, this stretch is ideal for anyone who could use more lower-leg flexibility.

1. Stand with toes of both feet about 12 to 18 inches (30 to 46 cm) from a wall.

2. Supporting yourself against the wall with one or both hands, take a big step back with your right foot,

keeping your left foot in place. Bending your left knee, keep your right leg straight with your heel flat on the ground to produce a gentle tug at the back of your lower leg (Achilles tendon) **a**. Hold and return to the starting position. Repeat on the other side.

TIP: Move your hips forward to increase the stretch.

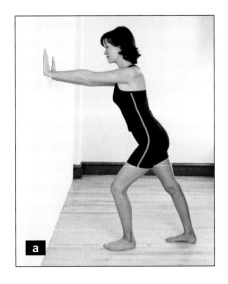

Seated Swivel

These moves give a more concentrated range-of-motion stretch to some of the muscles targeted by ankle circles, particularly those at the front and sides of your ankles.

1. Sit on the edge of a chair with feet flat on the floor about three to four inches (7.5 to 10 cm) apart.

2. Push up with your toes so that your heels rise off the floor. Turn your heels slowly and smoothly as far to the right as you comfortably can **a**. Hold.

3. Now turn heels slowly and smoothly to the left as far as you comfortably can **b**. Hold. Do this in both directions 6 to 8 times and return to the starting position.

4. Next, pull up with your toes so that they rise off the floor. Similar to the moves above, turn toes slowly and smoothly to the left and hold, then turn toes to the right and hold. Repeat 6 to 8 times.

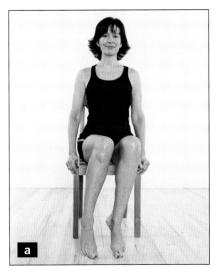

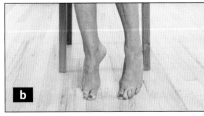

TIP: You may tend to swing your knees with the movement of this exercise, which is fine if it makes the motion more comfortable. As a rule, however, you'll get a better stretch if you keep your knees as steady as possible.

Toe Stretch and Curl

While sitting or standing, take your shoes off and simply stretch your toes apart as far as possible **a**. Try to wiggle your toes in as many directions as you can.

From a sitting or standing position with your shoes off, curl your toes as if you were trying to use your feet to grasp an object. Better yet, place a towel under your feet and repeatedly curl your toes to pull the towel closer **b**.

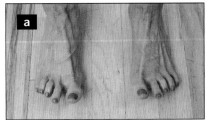

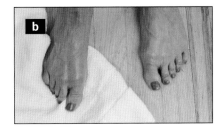

Ankles and Feet >

STRENGTH EXERCISES

LEVEL 1

Heel Raise

This exercise strengthens two major muscles in the calf and shores up the Achilles tendon.

1. Stand with your feet about hip-width apart, using a chair or wall to keep your balance.

2. Raise yourself on the balls of both feet so your heels lift off the floor as high as they comfortably can **a**. Slowly lower back to the floor.

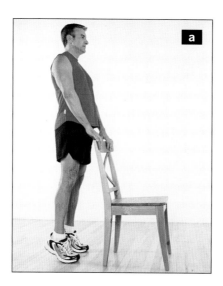

LEVEL 2

Stair Heel Raise

This exercise combines moves from the basic heel raises in level 1 and the stair calf stretches to work your calf and ankle muscles through a fuller (and more difficult) range of motion.

1. Stand on a stair with feet about hip-width apart, with your weight on the balls of your feet and your heels protruding over the edge of the stair.

2. Slowly lower your heels until you feel a stretch in your calves and the backs of your ankles **a**.

3. Lift your heels and stand as high on the balls of your feet as you comfortably can **b**. Hold for one second, then slowly lower to the starting position and repeat.

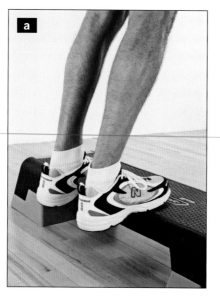
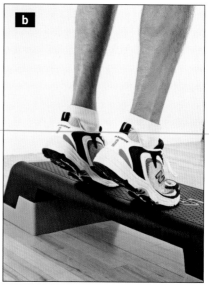

TIP: As with the stair calf stretch, be sure you stay under control through the entire motion, using a stair rail for support: Dropping heels suddenly below the level of the stair can overstretch the calves and strain the Achilles tendon.

Heel/Toe Raise

By combining two motions, this exercise works both the calves (when you're on the balls of your feet) and the muscles at the front of your shins (when you're on your heels).

1. Stand with both feet on the floor about hip-width apart using a chair, counter or wall for balance.

2. Rise up on the balls of your feet so that your heels come off the floor as far as comfortably possible **a**. Hold for one second and slowly lower your heels to the floor (the starting position).

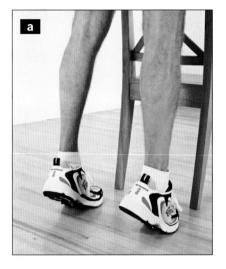 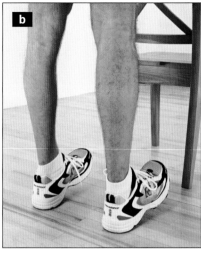

3. Elevate your toes and the front of your feet off floor as far as comfortably possible **b**. Hold for one second, then lower to floor to complete one repetition.

Ankle Roll

Doing this exercise may make you aware of muscles you didn't know you had—on the inside and outside of your ankles.

1. Sit in a chair with your feet flat on the floor about hip-width apart.

2. Using the muscles on the inside of your ankles, roll your feet outward along their outside edge so that the bottoms of your feet face toward each other **a**. Keeping your ankles moving, return to the starting position.

3. Using the muscles on the outside of your ankles, roll your feet along their inside edge so that the bottoms of your feet face away from each other **b**.

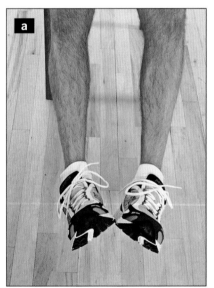 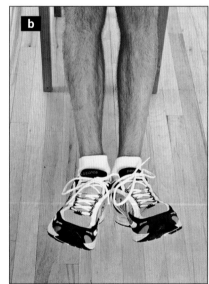

TIP: Concentrate on your ankle muscles as you do the exercise. These muscles should be producing the movement in your feet, not your knees or legs.

LEVEL 3

One-Foot Heel Raise

This is a variation on the heel raises in level 1, but it's more difficult because you stand on one foot instead of two.

1. Start with both feet flat on the floor about hip-width apart, then raise your left foot so it's just off the floor, putting all your weight on the right foot **a**. Hold a chair or counter for balance.

2. Raise yourself on the ball of your right foot so your heel lifts off the floor as high as comfortably possible **b**. Slowly lower back to the floor.

TIP: For an intermediate exercise that bridges two-foot and one-foot heel raises, do two-foot raises holding a light weight.

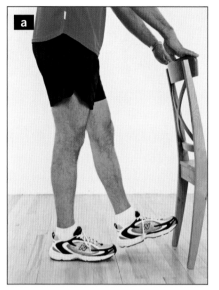

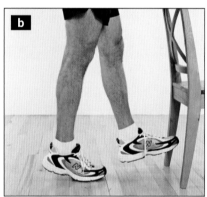

AT THE *Fitness Centre*

If you have access to good-quality exercise machines, here's what to use for your ankles and feet:

CALF PRESS MACHINE
If the design of the machine allows, position your feet on the plate so that your heels protrude off the edge, which grants a greater range of motion for this exercise.

MASSAGES

Foot Press

1. Place both hands across the top of your right foot, with your thumbs positioned next to each other on the bottom of the foot **a**.

2. Starting at the heel, use your thumbs to press into the bottom of the foot for one second, then release **b**. Inch your thumbs from your heel toward your toes, pressing and releasing as you go.

3. Do this twice on your right foot and repeat on the other foot.

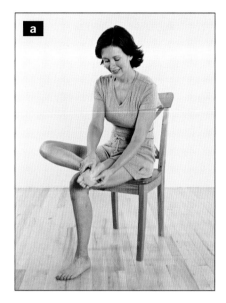
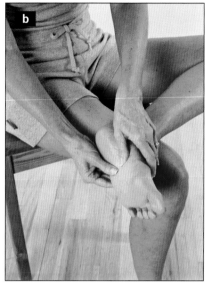

Foot Rocker

1. Start in the same position as the foot press, with hands across the top of your right foot and thumbs on the bottom **a**.

2. Squeeze your foot with your right hand and, while maintaining a firm grasp (not sliding or stroking), twist your hand forward, rotating the foot (The left hand should remain passive.) **b**. Now use the left hand to rotate the foot in the other direction while keeping the right hand passive. Do each motion twice and repeat on the other foot.

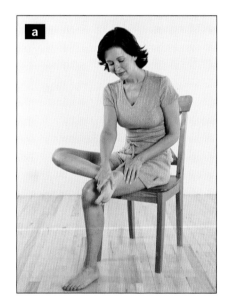
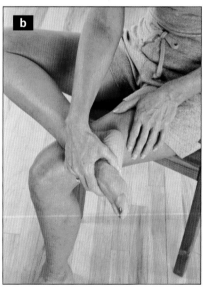

Toe Pull

1. Grasp the tip of your right big toe with the fingers of your left hand and gently pull on the toe while twisting the toe like a knob **a**.

2. Do this twice for each toe on your right foot and repeat on the other foot.

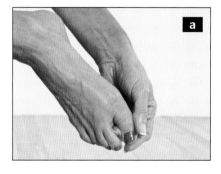

Though it's not as common to have arthritis in the elbows as in the hands, knees and hips, you shouldn't ignore the elbows, which are critically important for all the activities that involve the upper extremities. Increasing strength and flexibility in the elbows translates into improved ability to, say, get out of a chair or to pick up a grandchild. The elbow works with the shoulder and wrist to provide the entire arm with a wide variety of movements, especially if you work to increase its mobility and power.

STRETCHES

Arm Hang

This simple exercise is especially useful for improving mobility if you tend to keep elbows bent rather than extending your arms completely—common in people who have lost range of motion due to arthritis.

1. Stand straight with your feet hip-width apart and knees slightly bent.

2. Let your arms hang down by your side and try to straighten them as much as you comfortably can 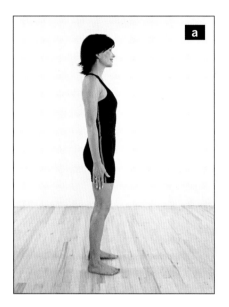. Stop the stretch just prior to locking your elbows. Hold.

TIP: You can also do this stretch while sitting straight on the edge of an armless chair.

Forearm Flip

1. Stand straight with your feet hip-width apart and knees slightly bent, arms hanging down by your side. Bend your elbows to 90 degrees with your palms facing upward as if you're holding a tray 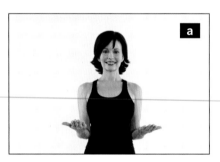. This is your starting position.

2. Smoothly flip your hands over so the palms are facing the floor as much as possible 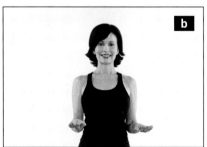. Hold and return to the starting position.

Shoulder Touch

Extending your thumbs in this exercise encourages you to provide more flexion to your elbows and helps keep your wrists properly aligned.

1. Stand straight with your feet hip-width apart and knees slightly bent, arms hanging down by your side, palms facing your thighs, fingers relaxed and thumbs pointing to the front **a**.

2. Smoothly bend your elbows, bringing your thumbs toward the same-side shoulders **b**. Hold. Slowly lower your hands back to the starting position.

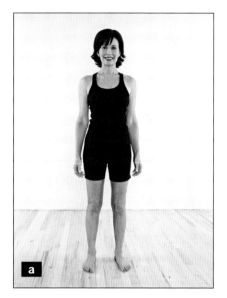

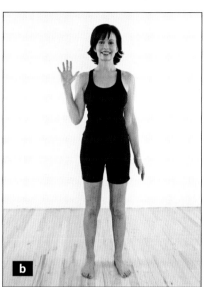

TIP: To maintain proper form, your elbows should remain next to your rib cage through the entire exercise.

STRENGTH EXERCISES

LEVEL 1

Seated Biceps Curl

This is a fundamental exercise for the biceps muscles that support the elbow at the front of the upper arm. It's a move that's easily adapted for different degrees of function and you'll find a variation in all three levels.

1. Sit up straight on the front half of an armless chair, feet flat on the floor, with your arms hanging down by your side **a**.

2. Smoothly bend your elbows, keeping them positioned at your side, raising your hands toward your shoulders while rotating your palms a quarter turn so they face your shoulder at the top of the movement **b**. Smoothly return to the starting position.

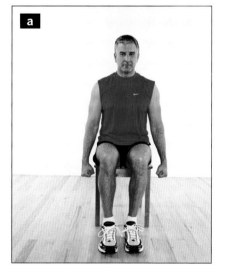

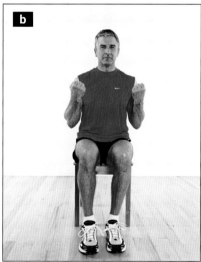

TIP: If you find it difficult or painful to lift your forearms from an extended position, rest your arm next to you on a table or the arm of a chair with your elbow padded by a towel as a starting position. This allows you to avoid the most difficult part of the movement while still working the biceps to increase strength. When you finish one arm, repeat with the other.

109

Armchair Dip

This is an exercise that encourages you to work muscles exactly the way you use them for everyday activities.

1. Sit in a sturdy armchair, back straight and feet flat on the floor about hip-width apart. Place your hands on the chair's arms about even with the front of your body **a**.

2. Using mostly your arms but assisting with your legs, push yourself out of the chair to a full standing position **b**, letting go of the chair as you stand **c**.

3. Lower yourself back into the chair, putting hands on the arms of

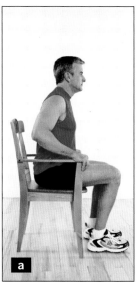 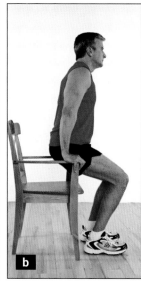 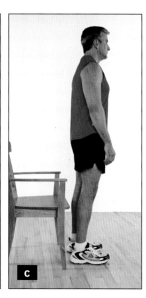

the chair as you slowly come down, using your arm muscles to return to the starting position.

TIP: For a variation maintain your hold on the arms of the chair until you fully extend arms then slowly lower yourself back into the chair.

LEVEL 2

Biceps Curl with Weights

This variation of the biceps curl adds hand weights for resistance. If you have trouble holding them, you can strap weights around your wrists for resistance.

1. Sit up straight on the front half of an armless chair, feet flat on the floor, your arms by your side and a hand weight in each hand **a**.

2. Slowly bend your right elbow, keeping it positioned at your side, raising the weight toward your shoulder while rotating your palm a quarter turn so it faces your shoulder at the top of the movement **b**.

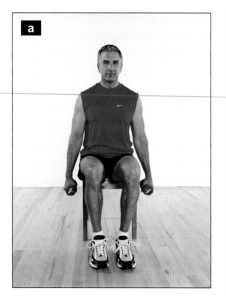 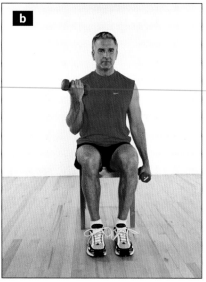

3. Slowly return to the starting position and repeat with the left arm for one repetition.

TIPS:
• Performing this exercise with alternating arms allows each arm to rest momentarily between repetitions.

• As you become stronger, do arms together. As that becomes easier, add weight and use alternating arms.

Hammer Curl

This exercise is similar to the standard biceps curl, but by angling the weight a different way, it also works muscles in the forearm that support the elbow.

1. Sit up straight on the front half of an armless chair, feet flat on the floor, arms hanging down by your sides and a hand weight in each hand, palms facing your thighs **a**.

2. Keeping your elbows close to your sides and your wrists straight, bend your right elbow, raising the weight end-first toward your right shoulder **b**.

3. Hold for one second and slowly return to the starting position. Repeat with the left arm.

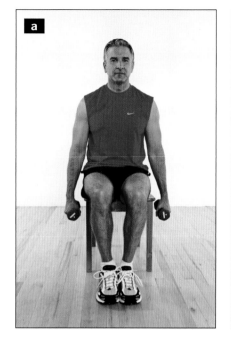

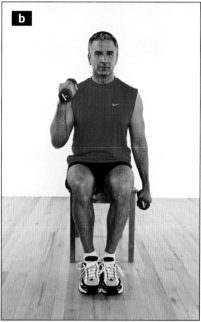

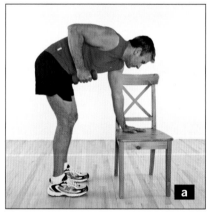

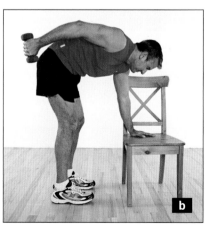

Triceps Kickback

This exercise works the muscles opposite the biceps on the back of your upper arm. If you have trouble holding hand weights, you can strap weights around your wrists for resistance.

1. Stand in front of a chair or bench holding a hand weight in your right hand. Bend forward at the waist, putting your left hand on the chair or bench so you feel stable. Keeping your knees slightly bent, bring your right elbow to your rib cage, so your arm is bent at about 90 degrees and the weight is hanging toward the floor **a**. This is your starting position.

2. Keeping your elbow next to your body, smoothly push the weight behind you, extending your elbow until it is nearly straight (but not locked) **b**.

3. Hold for one second and slowly lower the weight to the starting position. After completing one set, repeat with the left arm.

everyday
secrets

Leave the pool well. Finish off your water workout by using a fitness trick to get out of the pool. Go to the shallow end and stand with your back against the side of the pool. Reach back to place your palms on the edge of the pool and jump up so that you sit on the edge. Assisted by the buoyancy of your body in the water, this movement works your arms, shoulders, chest and back.

Park with employees. When shopping at the mall, park where workers are told to put their cars—away from entrances. Better yet, park at the end of the mall farthest from the store to which you're heading and walk to your destination. (Bonus: You'll have no trouble finding a spot.)

Take the long way. Most people try to find the shortest route to where they're going. But if you're hoofing it, short is good but long is better. Think of other ways to decide which way to go. Examples: Which way has more beautiful scenery, less traffic, a coffee shop, attractive stores or friendly people you might speak with?

continued on page 122

LEVEL 3

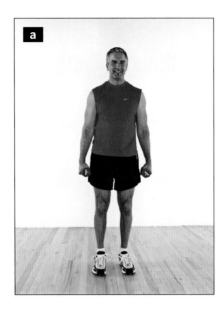

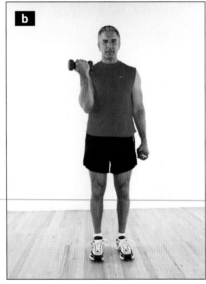

Standing Biceps Curl

By standing in this version of the biceps curl, you work your arm muscles but also call on muscles in the torso and lower body needed to stabilize your balance.

1. Stand straight with your feet hip-width apart and knees slightly bent, holding a hand weight in each hand with arms hanging down by your side, palms facing your thighs **a**.

2. Keeping your right elbow at your side, rotate your hand so your palm faces forward. Bend your elbow to raise the weight toward your shoulder so that your palm faces your shoulder at the top of the lift **b**.

3. Hold for one second and slowly lower the weight to the starting position, turning palms inward as you reach the bottom of the movement.

4. When your right arm is all the way down, repeat with the left arm.

TIP: It's tempting to come down only partway at the end of a biceps curl because the exercise becomes more difficult as your arm straightens. But it's important to bring arms all the way down and complete the wrist rotation at the bottom of every repetition. This momentarily works the biceps from a slightly different direction, making the exercise more effective.

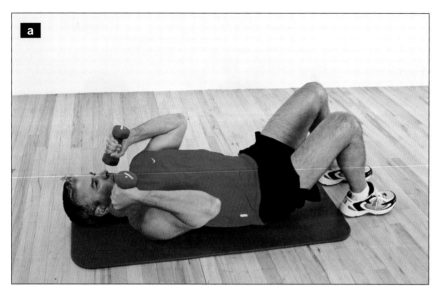

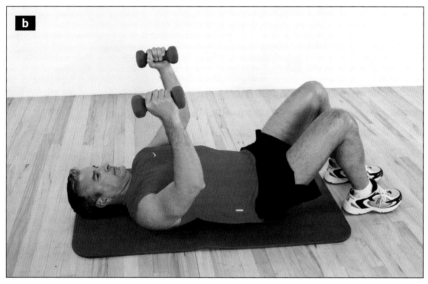

Lying Triceps Extension

1. Lie on the floor or an exercise mat with your knees bent and feet flat on the floor. Hold a hand weight in each hand, placing them vertically on end on the floor next to your ears **a**.

2. Keeping your elbows pointed toward the ceiling, straighten your arms as far as is comfortably possible without locking your elbows, so that knuckles will point toward the ceiling and the bars of the weights are parallel to the floor **b**.

3. Slowly lower the weight back to the floor to complete one repetition.

AT THE *Fitness Centre*

If you have access to good-quality exercise machines, here's what to use for your elbows:

SEATED TRICEPS PUSHDOWN
To effectively work your triceps muscles using this machine, lean forward slightly at the waist to put your body in a better-leveraged position.

ASSISTED DIP
When you press upward to straighten your arms, be sure that your elbows are not locked.

Wrists >

STRENGTH EXERCISES

LEVEL 1

Wrist Curl

This exercise works the wrist along with the entire forearm.

1. Sit in a chair with your forearms resting on your thighs and your hands extended off your knees with your palms facing upward. Relax your hands, allowing your fingers to drop toward the floor. This is your starting position **a**.

2. Slowly bend your wrists to bring your fingers up so they point toward the ceiling as far as is comfortably possible **b**.

3. Slowly lower your fingers back to the starting position for one repetition.

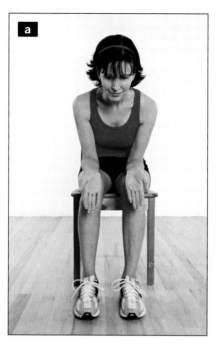

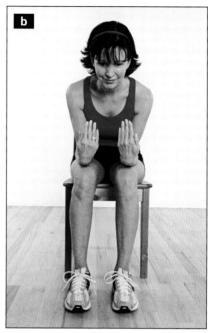

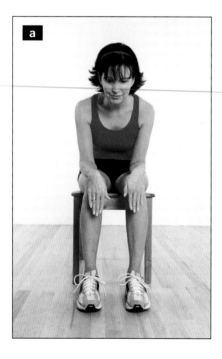

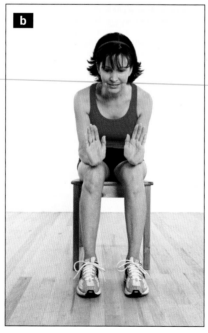

Wrist Extension

Think of this exercise as wrist curls in reverse.

1. Sit in a chair with forearms resting on your thighs and your hands extended over your knee with your palms facing the floor. Relax your wrist so your palms are against the upper part of your shin **a**.

2. Bending at the wrist, lift your hands upward as far as comfortably possible **b**.

3. Slowly lower your hands to the starting position and repeat.

Wrist Rotation

1. Sit in a chair, feet flat on the floor about hip-width apart. Rest your forearms on your thighs and extend your hands over your knees with your palms facing the floor.

2. Make loose fists **a** and, keeping your wrists straight, turn your fists so your palms are up **b**, Then turn them back so your palms are down again for one repetition.

TIP: You could also do this exercise with your hands open, but making a fist keeps the movement cleaner and prepares you for the level-2 version, in which you hold weights.

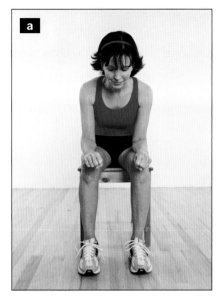
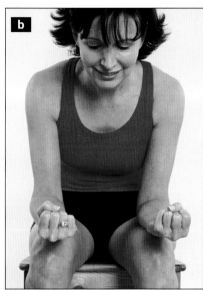

LEVEL 2

Weighted Wrist Curl

Performed like the wrist curls in level 1, this exercise is significantly more difficult with hand weights.

1. Sit in a chair holding a weight in each hand, with your forearms resting on your thighs and your hands extended off your knee with your palms facing upward. Relax your hands, allowing the weights to move toward the floor. This is your starting position **a**.

2. Roll your fingers to bring the weights comfortably into your hands. Slowly bend your wrists to bring the weights toward the ceiling as far as is comfortably possible **b**.

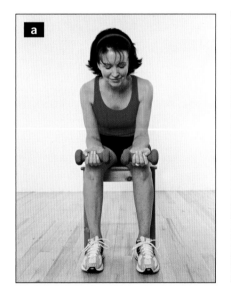
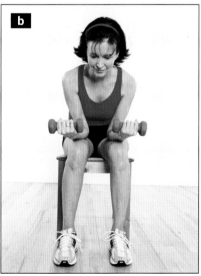

3. Slowly lower the weights back to the starting position for one repetition.

TIP: If you find it difficult to lift both weights together, start by doing alternating curls.

Wrists >

Weighted Wrist Extension

Here, too, the adding of hand weights makes this level-1 motion an exercise with level-2 intensity.

1. Sit in a chair and hold a weight in each hand, with forearms resting on your thighs and your hands extended over your knee with your palms facing the floor. Relax your wrists so the weights are resting against the upper part of your shins **a**.

2. Bending at the wrists, lift the weights upward as far as comfortably possible **b**.

3. Slowly lower your hands to the starting position and repeat.

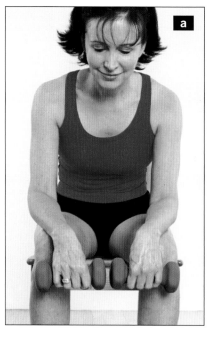

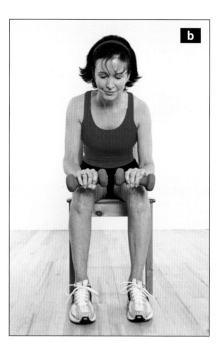

TIP: As with wrist curls, if you find it difficult to lift both weights together, start by alternating hands.

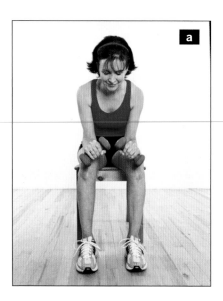

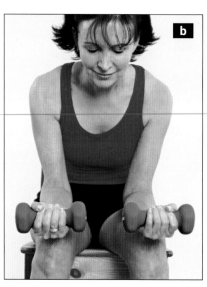

Weighted Wrist Rotation

Performed with hand weights, this exercise is more intense than the version in level 1.

1. Sit in a chair and hold a weight in each hand, forearms resting on your thighs, with palms facing downward and feet flat on the floor about hip-width apart.

2. Keeping your wrists straight, turn your fists **a** so your palms are up **b**, then turn them back so your palms are down again for one repetition.

TIP: If your weights tend to strike or get in each other's way, place your feet slightly farther apart to create more space between your knees.

LEVEL 3

Standing Wrist Curl

Though it's a curl, this exercise works at a more intense angle than regular curls, isolating muscles of the inner forearm.

1. Stand straight with your feet hip-width apart and your knees slightly bent. Grasp a hand weight in each hand, with your arms by your sides and palms facing behind you **a**.

2. Bend your wrist to curl your hands behind you as far as comfortably possible **b** **c**.

3. Slowly lower your hands to the starting position.

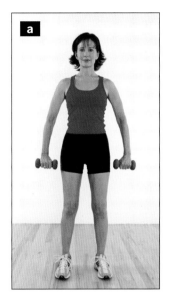
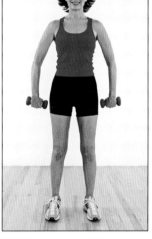
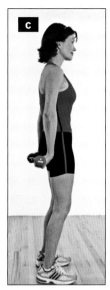

TIP: Before you try this exercise, be sure you can perform the backward-bending wrist movement without resistance to see if it causes any discomfort in your wrists, elbows or hands.

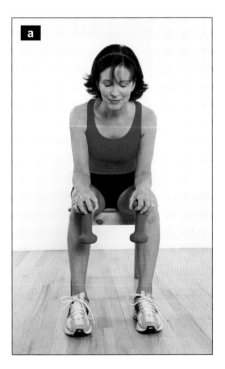
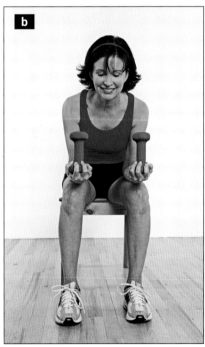

Thor's Hammer

Though the motion is similar to a wrist rotation, the way you hold the weights in this exercise adds consid-erably more resistance.

1. Sit in a chair and hold a weight in each hand, grasping the weight on one end (not in the middle of the handgrip) with palms facing downward **a**.

2. Keeping your wrists straight, turn the weights so your palms are up **b**. Then rotate hands back so your palms face down.

TIP: Start with a light weight—perhaps weighing 25 percent less than what you used for level-2 wrist curls. Or start with the lightest weight you have and work upward as your condition allows.

Hand joints are among the most common targets of arthritis. Yet because the muscles in the hands are small, you can give yourself a workout appropriate for restoring function with a minimal number of stretches and exercises involving very little resistance. What's more, exercises that you may already have done during your workout often do double duty working the hands. In fact, some of the best exercises for the hands involve movements that are also described in other sections.

STRETCHES

Finger Stretch

This is move is designed to extend your fingers' range of motion.

1. Place one hand on a tabletop or your thigh with your palm facing down.

2. Spread your fingers apart as far as you can and hold **a**. Repeat with the other hand.

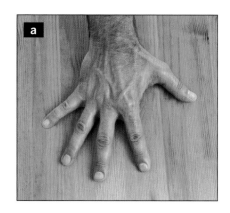

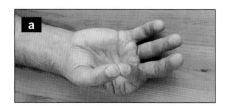

Gentle Fist

1. Place your right hand in a relaxed position, palm up, on a tabletop or your thigh.

2. Roll your fingers in toward your palm so that you make a loose fist. Try to bring your fingers as close together as is comfortable without squeezing **a**. Hold.

3. Release and roll your fingers out to the starting position and repeat with the other hand.

Thumb Touch

1. Place your hand, palm up, on a table with your fingers open and your hand relaxed.

2. Smoothly move the tip of your thumb into contact with the tip of your index finger, lightly touching, but not pressing them together **a**. Hold for one second. Relax and return to the starting position.

3. In a similar manner, bring your middle finger to your thumb, hold and return.

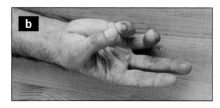

4. Do the same thing for the ring and pinkie fingers and repeat with the other hand **b**.

STRENGTH EXERCISES

LEVEL 1

Towel Grab

1. Lay a hand towel flat on a table-top. Place your right hand on the edge of the towel palm-down so that your fingers are on the edge of the towel, but the rest of your hand is off it **a**.

2. Slowly pull the towel toward the palm of your hand by bending all four fingers inward **b**. Continue for the entire length of the towel. Repeat with the other hand.

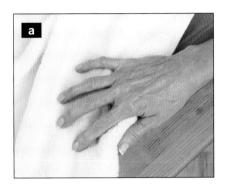
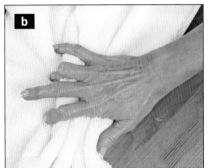

TIP: If arthritis pain or stiffness makes it difficult to pull a hand towel, start with a washcloth. To add resistance, the towel can be dampened with warm water.

Spider Walk

The movement in this exercise is a variation on the towel grab, but the weight of your arm provides more resistance.

1. Place your right hand palm-down on a tabletop **a**.

2. Using your fingers, pull your palms across the table as far as you can comfortably reach **b**. Repeat with the other hand.

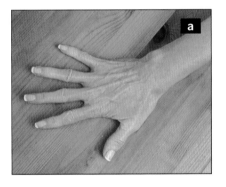
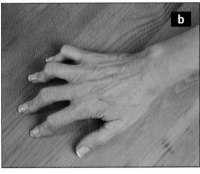

TIP: As you get stronger, add resistance by using fewer fingers to draw your hand across and alternate the exercise on different fingers to make sure each one gets a workout. Use as many or as few fingers as feels comfortable.

AT THE *Fitness Centre*

If you have access to good-quality exercise machines, here's what to use for your hands:

PULL-DOWN MACHINE
The reaching, grasping and pulling involved with this back exercise (see Back and Spine, page 86) make it an excellent exercise for the hands as well.

Wrist Curl

This exercise is good for the wrist (see also page 114), but uses the muscles of the hands to perform the movement.

1. Sit in a chair with your forearms resting on your thighs and your hands extended off your knees with your palms facing upward. Relax your hands, allowing your fingers to drop toward the floor. This is your starting position.

2. Slowly bend your wrists to bring your fingers up so they point toward the ceiling as far as is comfortably possible 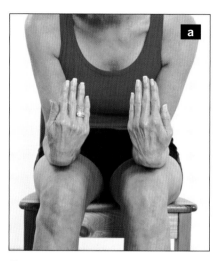.

3. Slowly lower your fingers back to the starting position for one repetition.

Wrist Extension

Another exercise that's described in the wrist section (see page 112), this movement also uses the muscles of the hands—but different ones from those used in wrist curls.

1. Sit in a chair with forearms resting on your thighs and your hands extended over your knee with your palms facing the floor. Relax your wrist so your palms are against the upper part of your shin.

2. Bending at the wrist, lift your hands upward as far as comfortably possible 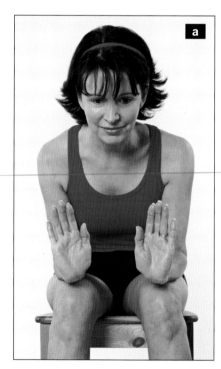.

3. Slowly lower your hands to the starting position and repeat.

MASSAGES

Palm Stroke

Hold your right palm facing up in your left hand so that your left thumb sits in your right palm 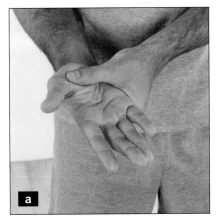. Press the flesh of your palm as you move your thumb in a straight line toward the base of your forefinger 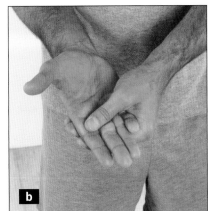. Do the same toward each finger. Do the entire exercise twice and repeat with the other hand.

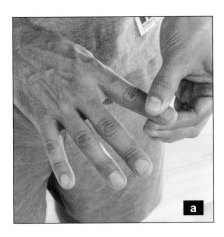

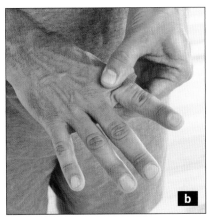

Finger Stroke

Take hold of your right forefinger with all the fingers of your left hand **a**. Starting from the middle knuckle, slide your fingers down the digit toward the base of the finger two times **a**. Then do the same thing from the fingertip to the middle knuckle **b**. Do this for all the fingers and repeat with the other hand.

Finger Twist

This massage increases both circulation and the motion of the joint.

1. As with finger strokes, take hold of your right forefinger with all the fingers of your left hand, as if you were putting on a ring.

2. Use the fingers of your left hand to twist the right finger like you're turning a knob, while sliding your fingers from the base of the digit to the fingertip **a**.

3. Do this twice for each finger and repeat on the other hand.

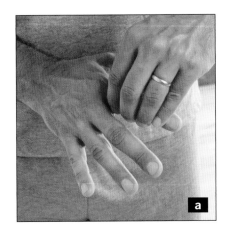

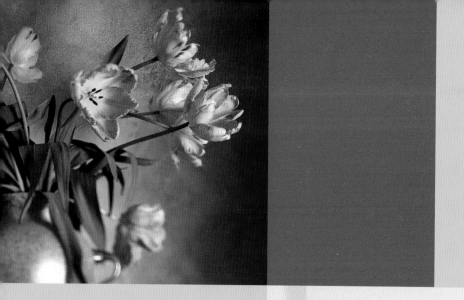

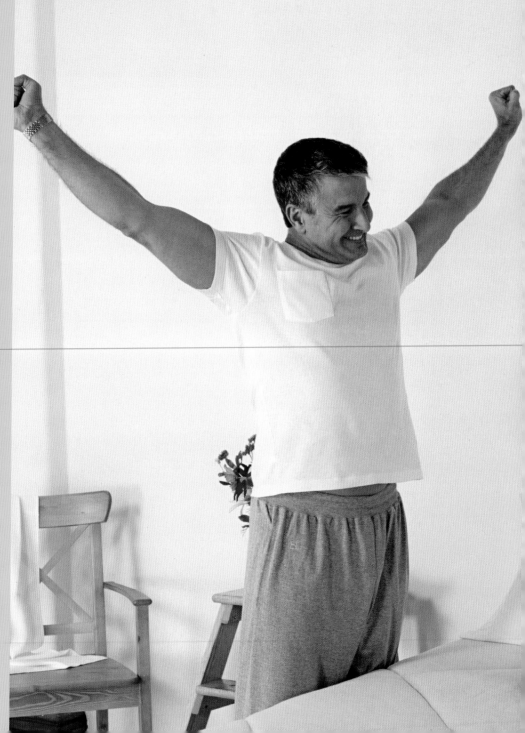

programs for living

Let's say you wanted to put together just five exercises or stretches that are best for you and you alone. Based on the exercises we just detailed in Part Three, you would have no less than 9 billion possible combinations! Clearly, you could use some help. ● The programs in this section are specifically designed to address some of the most common objectives of people with arthritis. Plus, we've put together more than 100 tips and secrets for easier living with arthritis.

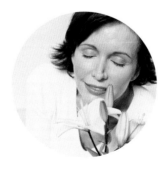

1 Easing Morning Stiffness

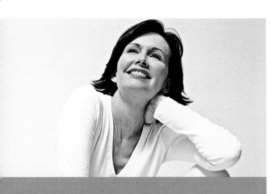

making the Program Work

Stretching and exercise don't have to be up-and-at-'em activities. This particular routine is gentle, calm, yet comprehensive, so that by the time your feet hit the floor, you've done a body-wide sequence of movements that will make it easier to carry on with your day. The exercises are designed to hit areas that are crucial for the mobility and dexterity you'll need to get through your morning routine. If you worry that your function level is lower in the morning than later in the day, rest assured that each of these stretches and exercises is appropriate for all but the most severe amounts of stiffness.

For many people with arthritis, mornings are the toughest time. Even after a restful night of sleep, the morning hours bring stiffness and pain.

For mornings like these, here is a gentle, eight-step exercise sequence to be done right in bed, right after you awaken.

Remember: No matter how much you wish to resist, moving your body is the best thing you can do. As you use joints and muscles, they loosen up and make the rest of your day easier. This routine, which mixes gentle stretches with simple strengthening moves, gives you an easy start that gradually makes further movement more manageable.

Instructions

For the stretches, hold your position for 15 seconds before releasing. For the strength exercises, do one set of 6 repetitions. Rest 30 seconds between each movement. Remain lying for the first three, then raise yourself to a sitting position for the rest. Move slowly and smoothly in a relaxed and gentle manner without a lot of abrupt motions. This ensures you'll gradually increase blood supply to stiff joints and supporting structures, warming them up and making them supple.

The Morning Routine

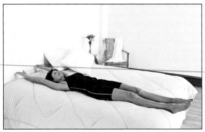

1. Lying Total Body Stretch

Without getting up, stretch your arms and legs to get blood flowing throughout your body. **Page 81**

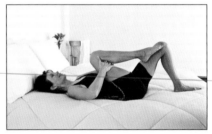

2. Low Back Knees to Chest

Push the covers off if you haven't already and slowly bring your knees to your chest. Return and repeat. This will help your back and hips. **Page 86**

Getting Out of Bed

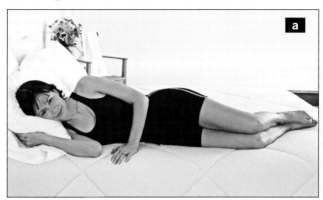

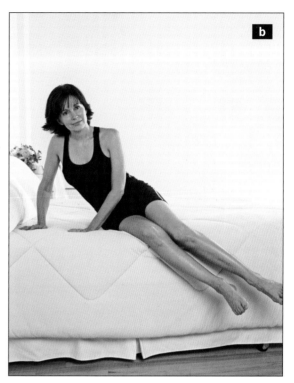

If back pain or other aches make getting out of bed in the morning a challenge, follow this technique.

1. First, roll onto your side, facing the edge of the bed **a**.

2. Next, swing your legs out over the edge. Then push your body up with your arms until you're in a sitting position on the edge of the bed **b**.

3. Finally, stand up solidly on both feet.

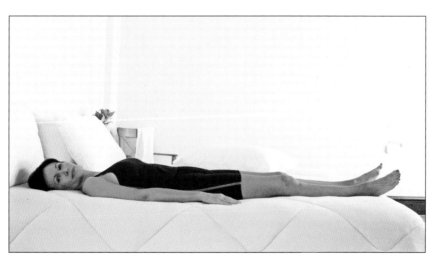

3. Neck Turn

While still lying down, gently stretch your neck muscles right and then left to ease tension in your head, neck and shoulders. **Page 98**

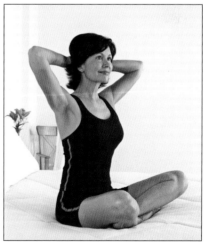

4. Seated Chest Stretch

Lengthen your chest muscles with this simple, pleasing stretch. **Page 94**

Program continues >   127

1 Easing Morning Stiffness

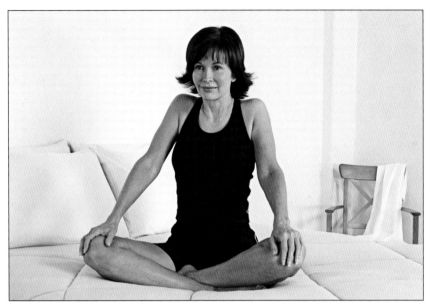

5. Shoulder Roll

Another soothing motion for your head, neck and shoulders. **Page 72**

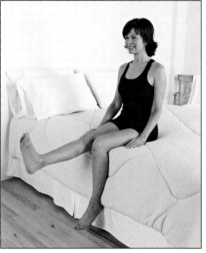

6. Seated Knee Extension

Slowly sit up for this stretch.
Page 56

everyday secrets

THE NIGHTTIME ROUTINE

Do a pre-sleep stretch. Stretching isn't just for the morning: Studies of patients with rheumatoid arthritis show that 15 minutes of stretching before you go to bed can significantly ease stiffness the next morning.

Prepare for nighttime nature calls. Make sure you clear a pathway to the bathroom that you can easily navigate in the dark before you go to bed. Keep doors fully opened or fully closed so you don't run into the edge. And even if you don't use a cane, walker or other assistance device during the day, consider keeping one by your bed at night to help ensure you keep your balance and detect obstacles when you're stiff and in the dark.

Take analgesics early. If you wake up early (perhaps to use the bathroom), take your pain-relieving medicine and go back to bed. This gives the drug time to kick in so that it's up to full strength when you actually get up to start your day.

Get hot in bed. If you have an electric blanket, turn up the heat just after waking to warm joints and help relieve morning stiffness.

Handle bed height. Mattresses today are much higher than in the past, which is a problem if it forces you to hop down from a height. Ways to manage meaty mattresses:

• Place a folding step stool with a handle next to the bed so you can climb down off the bed without putting extra strain on your joints.

• Get a platform bed that requires just a mattress, eliminating the extra height of a box spring.

Don comfy clothes. Putting on an extra layer of clothing as soon as you get out of bed may help you warm your joints faster. A sweatshirt and sweatpants would be a good bet, but if you find it difficult to pull them on, try putting on a fleece vest or a sweatshirt that zips. Another option: a bathrobe made of thick terry cloth, chamois or wool.

Choose practical slippers. Slippers without a back are easier to get in and out of than heel-covering styles. But backless slippers are more difficult to keep on when going up and down stairs.

THE MORNING ROUTINE

Get a grip. The trick to taking the discomfort out of manipulating thin toothbrush handles is to beef up the grip. Ways to make your oral hygiene more effective:

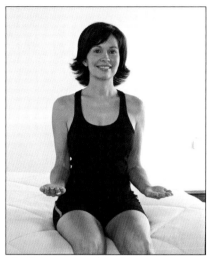

7. Forearm Flip

Now give your elbows some relief and exercise with this gentle movement. **Page 108**

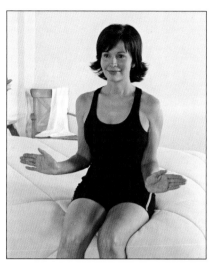

8. Wrist Circle

End the sequence with these gentle moves to ready your hands and wrists for washing, brushing your teeth and preparing breakfast. **Page 115**

ENTER THE SHOWER SAFELY

The best bet for getting in and out: Use a shower stall instead of a bathtub, which allows you to simply walk into the shower without lifting your legs over the edge of a tub. But when dealing with a tub, start by getting in at the end farthest from the faucet or shower head, which is likely to be a bit drier, warmer and less slippery. Stand with your hip to the side of the tub, bend the knee closest to the tub, keeping your upper leg straight so that you raise your foot behind you, then swing your foot into the tub and bring your other foot over the same way.

• Wrap your toothbrush in slip-on grips, spongy tape or other materials that hardware or medical specialty stores may offer to make handles thicker. Ad hoc alternative: Wrap handles in foam hair curlers or a sponge.

• Get an electric toothbrush, which will have a thick plastic handle (where batteries are typically stored) and doesn't require vigorous hand motion to give your teeth a thorough cleaning.

Tackle toothpaste. When painful, stiff or weak hands make squeezing the toothpaste tube difficult, let your fingers off the hook. Put the tube down on the counter and lean on it gently with the heel of your palm or even your elbow to squeeze out a small amount of paste and apply it to your brush.

Focus on fixtures. Ease discomfort from turning on the water by installing handles that extend and can be grabbed with your entire hand rather than compact handles that must be twisted with your fingers.

Manage medicine lids. If there are no children or grandchildren in the house, ask your pharmacist to fill your prescription using non-childproof lids, which screw or lift off like they did in the old days. If kid safety is an issue, ask a family member or friend to help sort your medications into a weekly dispenser with a handy flip-top compartment containing pills for each day of the week.

Take a shower. The heat and rush of water soothe joints and muscles and help your whole body relax, so it's important that the bath or shower itself doesn't become more of an obstacle or source of discomfort than necessary. Basic arthritis-friendly fixtures for easier, safer bathing include:

• Nonskid bath mats to provide sure footing both in the tub or shower stall and the neighbouring tile floor. As an added precaution, you can also wear the grip-soled water shoes you may already have for a pool exercise class.

• Bars you can grab to keep your balance and push or pull on while getting in or out.

• A shower seat where you can sit if you get fatigued. If there's not one built into the shower, consider using a folding beach chair or campstool.

• A handheld shower nozzle that can direct water at any angle. If you have a nozzle installed, have the plumber put it at waist height so it's easy to lift on and off. ■

2 Total Body Stretch

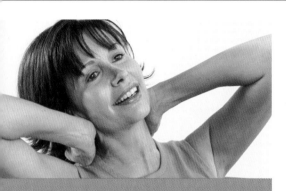

It's tempting just to stretch muscles supporting joints that hurt. But taking that approach would be a mistake. Good flexibility is something *every* joint needs for greater mobility and better posture. Plus, stretched muscles ease tension and take pressure off joints throughout your body.

This program is designed to improve body-wide flexibility with a mix of stretches that hit all your major joints and muscles. Don't be daunted by the 14-stretch sequence. Each exercise takes 15 to 60 seconds, so you can easily do this entire routine in just 5 to 10 minutes, plus a warmup.

Instructions

Begin with 5 to 10 minutes of easy walking or some other light activity to warm up your muscles, tendons and ligaments. This makes stretches both safer and more effective. Perform the stretches as described in Part III, holding each stretch according to the guidelines for your function level. Flow from one stretch to the other without much pause.

making the
Program Work

It's not harmful to do these stretches in a different order or to make substitutions for any that feel uncomfortable. But going through the program as outlined has a number of benefits. The idea is to start with a gentle movement that stretches the entire body all at once, then proceed from larger muscles or groups of muscles to smaller or more isolated ones.

The program also keeps exercises moving from one area of the body to another so that stretching activity is evenly distributed as you go. Stretches for muscles that tend to be less pliable in most people (such as the hamstrings in the seated V) are placed so that easier stretches can first prep the area with some preliminary limbering. The workout finishes with a posture exercise that will keep you standing tall even as you move on with your day.

The Stretch Sequence

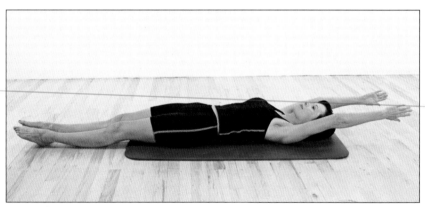

1. Lying Total Body Stretch

This stretch feels great and expands your whole body. It is particularly good for your shoulders and abdomen. **Page 81**

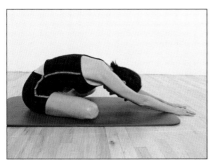

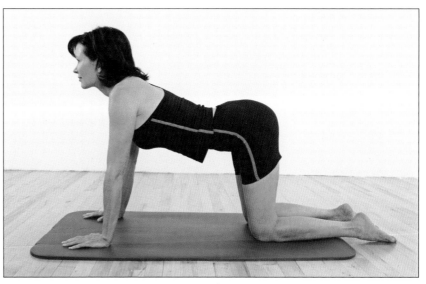

2. Cross-Legged Seated Stretch

Sit up now for a soothing stretch that benefits your lower back. **Page 88**

3. Cat Stretch

Gently pull yourself forward onto your hands and knees for another great stretch for your back. **Page 88**

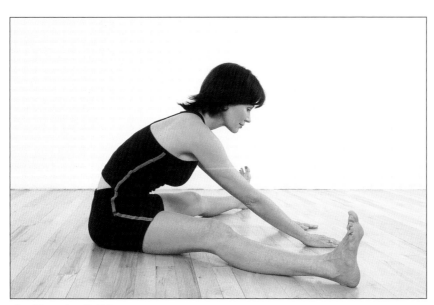

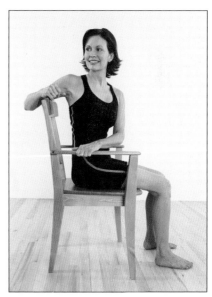

4. Seated V

Now plop back down on your butt, stretch your legs out in front of you and reach! This stretch helps your knees, hips and back. **Page 57**

5. Seated Torso Twist

In a chair, stretch your abdomen muscles for better posture and back support. **Page 80**

Program continues >

2 Total Body Stretch

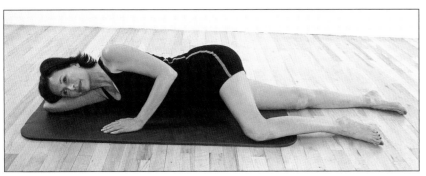

6. Lying Pelvis Rotation

Relax onto the ground and give your hips some relief with this gentle torso stretch. **Page 59**

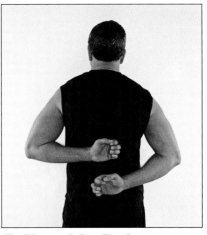

7. Knuckle Rub

Now to your upper body: Work out the tension in your shoulder and neck muscles. You should feel this one deeply. **Page 73**

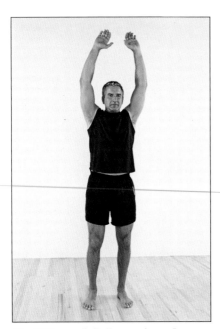

8. 'Good Morning' Exercise

Say hello to the world with this soothing shoulder stretch. **Page 74**

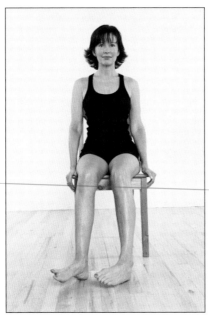

9. Ankle Circle

Gentle foot rotations will help your ankles cope with the day's travels. **Page 102**

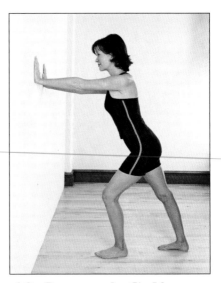

10. Runner's Calf Stretch

This popular stretch does wonders for that important muscle that connects your knee to your ankle. **Page 103**

everyday
secrets

STRETCHING

Breathe deep. Make your stretching even more relaxing and pain relieving by working in elements of meditation. Specifically, try these simple breathing techniques:

• Breathe through your nose both when inhaling and exhaling.

• Focus on the hiss of air flowing in and out of your nostrils; the calming tone soothes your thoughts.

• Take at least three seconds to fill your lungs and another three to let air out.

Unclench your stretch. Stretching should relax all of you. Don't let your jaw, shoulders, hands and feet tense up during your routine. Tense body parts make stretching other areas less effective.

Get an extra stretch. The rule of thumb is to stretch until you feel a gentle tug in the muscle. But if that feeling subsides as you hold, are you stretching far enough? The answer is yes—for the 15 seconds or so it takes your muscles to relax with the stretch. That might be enough for you. But if you feel limber enough to push a little farther, stretch another fraction of an inch after you've held for 15 seconds,

then hold for another 15 seconds. This extra push, sometimes called the developmental stretch, helps promote flexibility faster than the first stretch alone.

Keep it up. Even if you don't do other aerobic or strength exercises, it's worth stretching every day: Lengthened muscles only keep their newfound flexibility for a day or less. Consistently working them every day, however, makes them progressively more pliable—as long as you keep stretching. Plus, stretching is good for stress relief and your attitude—every day. ■

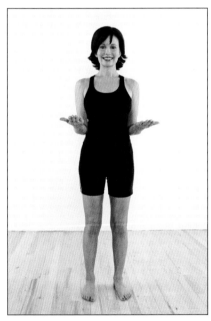

11. Forearm Flip

Almost done. Now do this gentle but important stretch for your elbow. **Page 108**

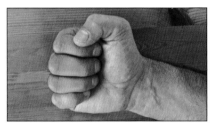

12. Gentle Fist

Bring blood into those fingers and stretch those hand muscles with this simple, reflexive movement. **Page 120**

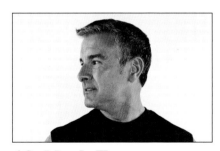

13. Neck Turn

Amazing how much tension finds its way into your neck muscles. These turns offer quick relief. **Page 98**

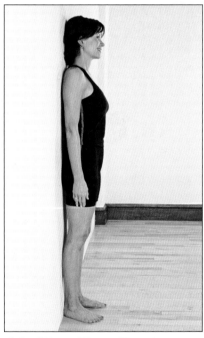

14. Standing Posture Exercise

Conclude this refreshing sequence with a slow, energizing stretch for the spine. **Page 86**

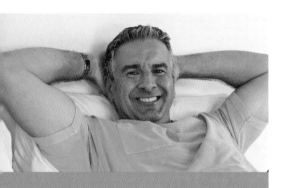

Imagine a strength-training workout that only exercised your arms. You'd find it easy to lift groceries out of the trunk—

but if your legs were weak, you'd have trouble hauling the load up the stairs. Exercise needs to be balanced to make sure your whole body—not just one part—becomes stronger and more mobile. While selected exercises can bolster specific joints, it's important to establish a foundation of strength in all your major muscles that targeted workouts can build upon.

making the
Program Work

The basic pattern of a strength workout is to alternate exercises between upper and lower extremities, the front and back of the body or pushing and pulling motions—all of which allow freshly-worked muscles to rest while you hit another area. As you progress through the workouts, you generally go from larger muscles or groups of muscles to smaller ones, with abdominal exercises in the middle to break things up. While each workout targets all the major muscles, a greater number of exercises are devoted to the lower body, which has more muscles that are critical for overall mobility.

Instructions

You will find three different routines on the following pages: beginning, intermediate and advanced. On page 55, we give details on how to increase the challenge within each routine as you get stronger. And when you feel like you've mastered one routine, proceed to the next! For each exercise listed, do the following number of repetitions the first time you attempt the program.

■ **Beginning:** Do one set of six repetitions.

■ **Intermediate:** Do one set of six to eight repetitions.

■ **Advanced:** Do one set of eight repetitions.

■ BEGINNING Strength Program

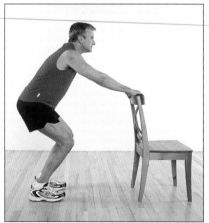

1. Partial Squat

Start your workout with this simple exercise for the hips and thighs. **Level 1, page 61**

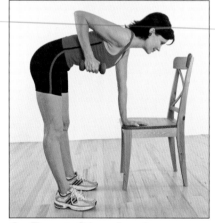

2. Bent Single Arm Row

It would seem like this is an arm exercise, but it is your back muscles doing the work. **Level 2, page 92**

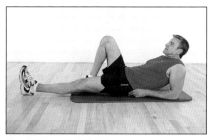

3. Heel Slide

Back to your lower body with this exercise for knees and hips.
Level 1, page 62

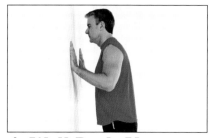

4. Wall Push-Up

This stand-up alternative to the classic exercise is a great way to gently strengthen your chest.
Level 1, page 95

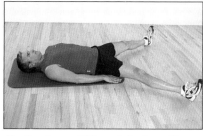

5. Lying Hip Abduction

Get out your mat and on your back to give some exercise to your hips. **Level 1, page 61**

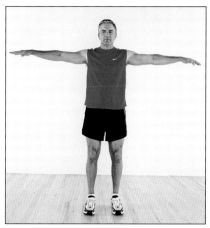

6. Around the World

Get your shoulders moving gently and steadily for suppleness and strength. **Level 2, page 78**

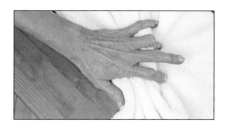

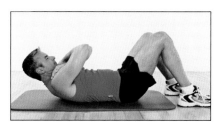

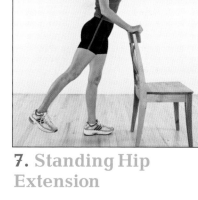

7. Standing Hip Extension

Your hip muscles just got a rest; let's get them moving again.
Level 2, page 64

9. Towel Grab

Can't forget the hand and finger muscles. Do 2 repetitions of this exercise with a 30-second break in between reps. **Level 1, page 121**

10. Basic Abdominal Curl

Down one more time for this classic exercise. If it's too tough, do the level 1 modified curl instead.
Level 2, page 82

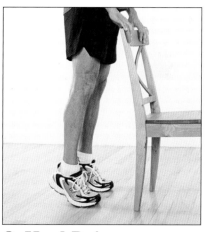

8. Heel Raise

Now exercise your ankles and feet. **Level 1, page 104**

3 Total Body Strength

■ INTERMEDIATE Strength Program

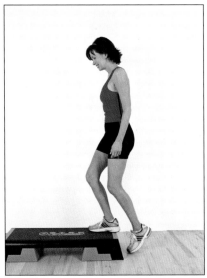

1. Stair Step-Up

Six to eight of these on each side will give your knees and hips a good workout. **Level 2, page 65**

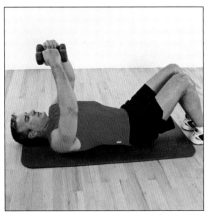

2. Weighted Chest Fly

As your legs rest, here is a great exercise for your chest muscles. **Level 2, page 96**

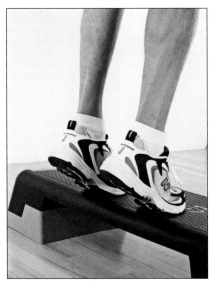

3. Stair Heel Raise

Back to your step for this subtle but useful exercise for ankles and feet. **Level 2, page 104**

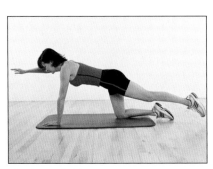

4. Bird Dog

Down on the floor now for this natural strengthener for hips and back. **Level 2, page 66**

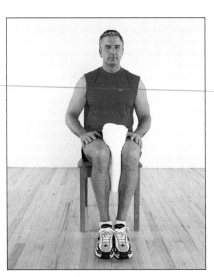

5. Towel Squeeze

It seems so simple, but this exercise really does strengthen your hips. **Level 1, page 62**

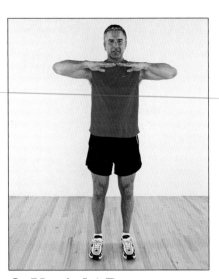

6. Upright Row

Another natural move that, when done in repetition, builds up muscles. **Level 2, page 77**

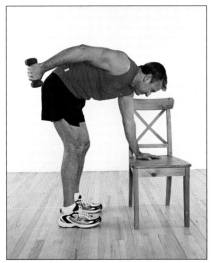

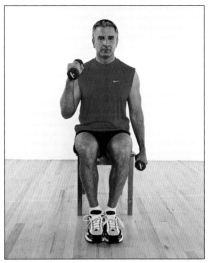

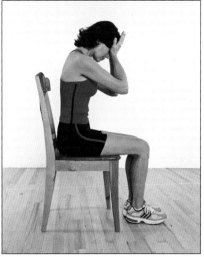

7. Triceps Kickback

Triceps don't get much exercise, so be ready for the challenge!
Level 2, page 111

8. Hammer Curl

The classic exercise for bigger biceps is also wonderful for your elbow. **Level 2, page 111**

9. 'Yes' Exercise

This agreeable exercise is great for your neck (and your attitude). **All levels, page 99**

Program continues >

everyday *secrets*

STRENGTHENING

Book yourself. Don't have time for all this exercise? Sometimes it's a matter of perception—other people's. If co-workers, friends or even family can't understand why you take time for exercise but not for what they think is important, keep your priorities to yourself—but schedule your exercise in your date book. That way, when sticking to your guns on workouts, you can merely say you're keeping a prior appointment.

Keep it interesting. Some people have a high tolerance for routine—and may even elevate it to ritual. But if your attention span is closer to monkey than monk, try to introduce variety into your workout on a regular basis. One way to do it: Change two things about your routine every week. It could be as simple as adding repetitions, resistance or sets—or substituting one exercise for another. Change isn't just an antidote to boredom, it allows you to continually challenge muscles in new ways, which makes you stronger faster.

Try slow motion. Want to try a difficult challenge that's easy on joints? Lift a light weight only one time—but do it very slowly. Pick out a weight about half what you'd normally lift 10 times. Take 15 to 20 seconds to lift the weight, hold for another 15 to 20 seconds, then take another 15 to 20 seconds to bring it back down. The constant stress through the entire range of motion will work muscles in an entirely new way.

Judge gym transit time. Made the decision to join a health club? When choosing, follow the golden rule of gym location: Keep it within a 15-minute drive. Any farther and your chances of actually getting there for a workout drop considerably.

Spread the effort. If doing an entire full-body workout all at once is too fatiguing or demanding on your time, try doing only one part of the workout each day. If your workout has 12 exercises,

continued on page 140

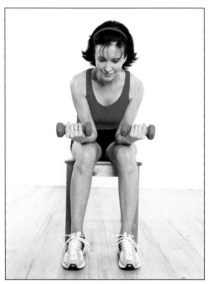

10. Weighted Wrist Curl

This small move is harder than you'd expect, since we rarely test our forearm muscles. **Level 2, page 117**

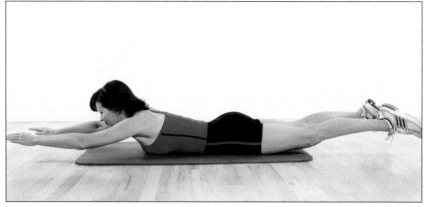

11. Superman

Another feel-good exercise, this time for a healthier and stronger back.
Level 2, page 91

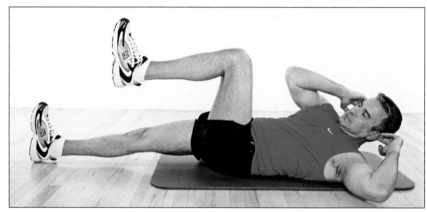

12. Basic Bicycle

End your workout with this youthful move for your abdomen. **Level 2, page 83**

AS YOU GET STRONGER

Here is how to progress as you get better with your exercises:

■ When you feel comfortable doing the number of starting repetitions, add no more than 1 repetition each time you work out. For example, if you start with 1 set of 6 reps, you could do 1 set of 7 reps next time—or stay at 6 reps if that's still challenging.

■ Advance by adding 1 repetition at a time until you can do 12 reps of upper-body exercises and 15 of lower-body exercises. Continue with that number for two or three consecutive workouts.

■ In your next workout, do 1 set of 8 repetitions, rest one to two minutes, then do a second set of 8 repetitions for a total of 16 repetitions. Alternative:

increase the amount of weight (in non-body-weight exercises where you can adjust resistance) by the smallest amount possible (probably 1 pound) and go back to the number of starting reps.

■ Continue progressing, changing either the number of sets or amount of resistance (but not both at once) as you go get stronger.

■ ADVANCED Strength Program

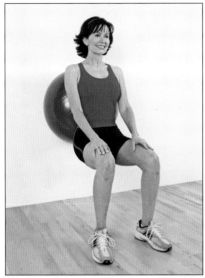

1. Ball Squat

If you don't have an exercise ball, do regular squats. **Level 3, page 67**

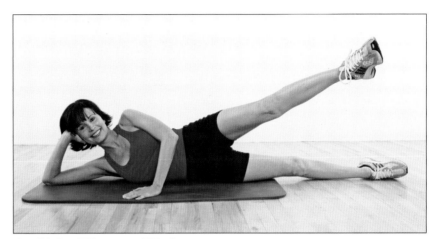

2. Side Thrust Kick

This challenges a different set of leg muscles, but aids those same knees and hips. **Level 3, page 67**

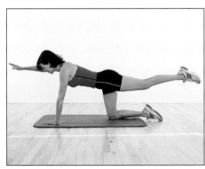

3. Advanced Bird Dog

S-t-r-e-e-e-t-c-h and strengthen your hips and back with this fun exercise. **Level 3, page 93**

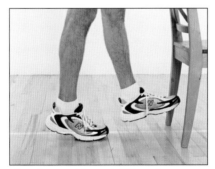

4. One-Foot Heel Raise

Strengthen your ankles and feet and improve your balance with this one. **Level 3, page 106**

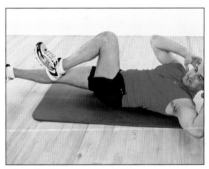

5. Advanced Bicycle

This abdominal muscle builder will help you transition from lower- to upper-body exercises. **Level 3, page 85**

Program continues >

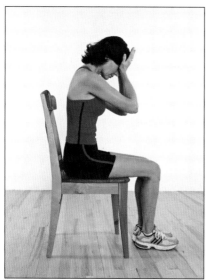

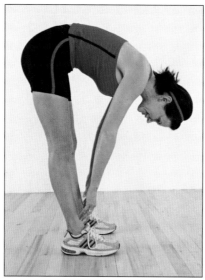

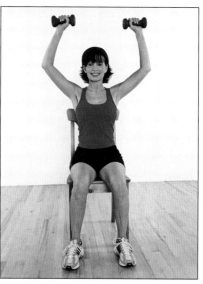

6. 'Yes' Exercise

Not as strenuous, but still an important strengthener for the often-neglected neck muscles. **All levels, page 99**

7. Dead Lift

An Olympic-level test! But for you, go slow, easy and smooth for a better back. **Level 3, page 92**

8. Overhead Dumbbell Press

Another classic exercise for strength builders, this for your shoulders. **Level 3, page 79**

continued from page 137

for example, do the first three on Monday, the next three on Tuesday and the rest on Wednesday. On Thursday, start the routine again. That way, you're still doing each exercise three times during a one-week period without exhausting yourself with your routine.

Hold on to your gains. While giving your muscles a chance to rest is important to making them stronger, there's inevitably a point of diminishing returns when it comes to slacking off. How much rest is too much? A good rule of thumb is to expect about a 10 percent loss of your strength gains after about 10 days. The more training you've done, the slower your strength will decline. The bottom line: To maintain your gains, you need to keep exercising regularly.

Count backward. Problem: Strength exercises are no fun when the last repetitions are tough to do. Interpretation: If you're challenging your muscles enough to want to quit, you're probably doing them at just the right intensity. Mental trick: Your final repetitions will seem easier if you count backward from your target instead of forward from zero because you'll be thinking about how few you have left, rather than how many you've already done.

Get off the floor safely. For exercises and stretches that require you to get on all fours, it's easier to get back up again if you walk your hands back until you're in a kneeling position, place one foot on the floor in front of you with your knee bent at about 90 degrees, then use your leg as a support for your hands as you stand or ease yourself into a chair. ■

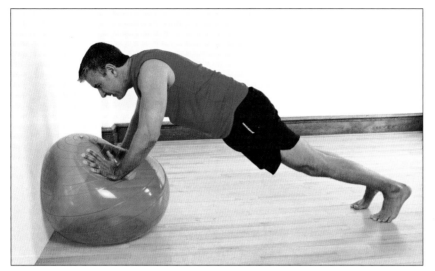

9. Ball Push-Up

A great exercise for your chest. Feel proud if you can do eight good ones. **Level 3, page 97**

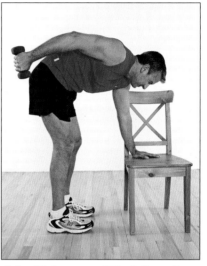

10. Triceps Kickback

It looks so simple and natural, but this arm exercise can be challenging. **Level 2, page 111**

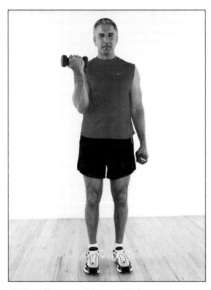

11. Standing Biceps Curl

Don't think about your biceps; think about a better-supported elbow joint. **Level 3, page 112**

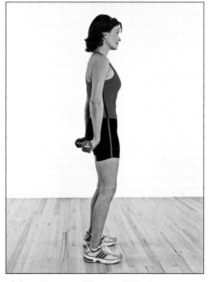

12. Standing Wrist Curl

End this strengthening routine with this simple move for healthier wrists and hands. **Level 3, page 119**

AT THE FITNESS CENTRE

Want a total strengthening program using the machines at the health centre? These are the 12 exercises we recommend. Start with two sets of six repetitions of each and work up from there. Do in the order listed:

1. Leg Press
2. Knee Flexion
3. Machine Abduction/Adduction
4. Pull-Down
5. Chest Press
6. One-Foot Heel Raise
7. Machine Overhead Press
8. Standing Biceps Curl
9. Seated Triceps Pushdown
10. Weighted Wrist Extension
11. Ball Curl
12. Weighted Wrist Rotation

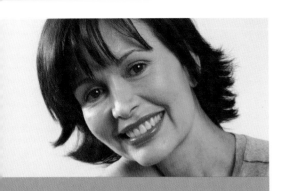

making the
Program Work

There's a reason why you need both cardiovascular (aerobic) exercise and strength training to effectively lose weight. The aerobic exercise burns lots of calories *while* you exercise. And strength training causes more calories to be burned *after* you exercise. The reason: Muscle tissue is hungrier for energy than other types of tissue, especially fat.

In the aerobic program, progress at your own pace using perceived exertion as the primary measure of your progress. Although the cardio program is designed with walking in mind, you can use the same guidelines for other aerobic activities such as bicycling or swimming.

It's enough of a challenge to carry groceries from the car. But what if you were hauling weight that you could never put down?

That's the dilemma of being overweight when you have arthritis. Carrying extra pounds puts constant pressure on joints that subjects them to more stress and contributes to pain.

Losing weight requires that your body burn more energy (calories) than you take in. That makes a good diet half of the equation. The other half, exercise, works in two essential ways. First, you burn calories through your activity. But second, you also boost your metabolism—both during your workout and for as long as 24 to 48 hours later! By keeping a regular schedule of exercise, you'll perpetually boost your calorie-burning metabolism and keep notching it higher as you go.

Instructions

There are two parts to this program: Aerobic routines and strength-building exercises. Follow the aerobic program described on page 146. It asks for you to take walks four to six days per week, so be prepared for some pleasant outdoor time!

As for strengthening, we've given you three programs to choose from: beginning, intermediate and advanced. On page 138, we give details on how to increase the challenge within each program as you get stronger. And when you feel like you've mastered one routine, proceed to the next! For each exercise listed, do the following number of repetitions the first time you attempt the program.

■ **Beginning:** Do one set of six repetitions.

■ **Intermediate:** Do one set of six to eight repetitions.

■ **Advanced:** Do one set of eight repetitions.

The strength-training programs we created have four unique weight-loss benefits:

1. They focus on building large muscles, which tend to use more energy;

2. They were chosen with the functional limits of an overweight person in mind;

3. Most of the exercises use multiple joint movements to involve as many muscles as possible;

4. They are sequenced to keep your body moving through different positions to burn even more calories.

■ BEGINNING Strength Program

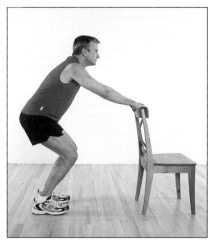

1. Partial Squat

Start with this simple exercise for your hips and knees; use the chair for balance and safety. **Level 1, page 61**

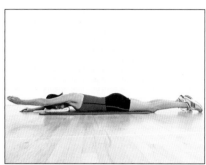

2. Lying Alternating Arm Raise

Off your feet for this exercise that, surprisingly, is for your back, not your arms or shoulders. **Level 1, page 90**

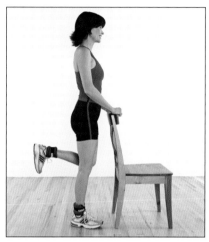

3. Standing Knee Flexion

And now back up (that's part of the exercise!) and do this exercise to strengthen your leg muscles and support your hip and knee. **Level 2, page 64**

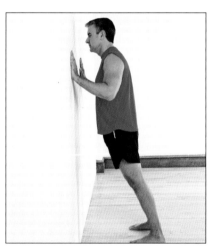

4. Wall Push-Up

Strengthening your chest muscles helps you breathe better and lift easier. **Level 1, page 95**

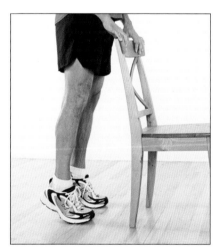

5. Heel Raise

This seems like such a simple move, but it does wonders for your feet, ankles and lower legs. **Level 1, page 104**

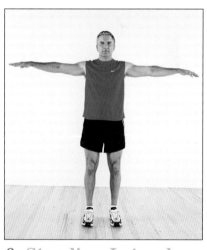

6. Standing Lateral Raise

Another very natural move— lifting your arms!—but a good workout for your shoulder muscles and joints when done in repetition. **Level 2, page 77**

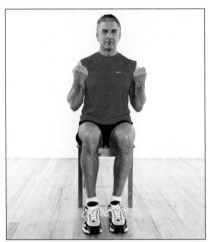

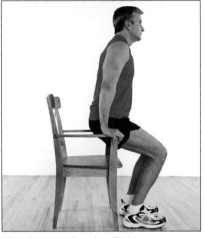

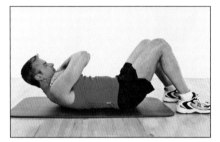

7. Seated Biceps Curl

The classic weightlifting move! But strong biceps aren't just for show—they make carrying things easy and support your elbow. **Level 1, page 109**

8. Armchair Dip

Behind the biceps muscle is the triceps. This exercise strengthens that muscle and also aids your elbows. **Level 1, page 110**

9. Basic or Advanced Abdominal Curl

Remember: Abs exercises don't reduce abdominal fat. But strong abs support your back and make lifting easier. **Level 2 or 3 depending on variation, page 82 or 84**

everyday *secrets*

BURNING CALORIES

Get on the vacuum program. Make vacuuming a total body exercise by stepping forward in a slightly longer-than-usual stride as you move the carpet machine forward while keeping your back straight, then stepping back as you draw the unit toward you again. At the same time you work the muscles of your legs with this lunge-like motion, roll the vacuum cleaner forward with your arms, which uses your shoulder, chest, arm and upper back for a near-complete workout that contains elements of both strength and aerobic conditioning.

Make every movement count. Fidgeting burns hundreds of calories a day, according to studies at the Mayo Clinic in Rochester, Minnesota and even chewing gum eats up 11 calories an hour. So don't lose sight of the fact that any form of physical activity—no matter how small—helps your body burn calories. More ways to get movement into your everyday life:

• Always stand up and walk around when on the telephone.

• Always stand up and walk around during television commercials.

• Chop your vegetables by hand, rather than using a food processor.

• While in the car, roll your shoulders and stretch your arms at red lights.

■ INTERMEDIATE Strength Program   Starting point: 1 set of 6 to 8 repetitions.

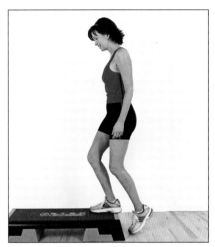

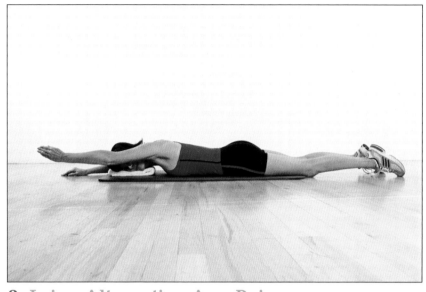

1. Stair Step-Up

By strengthening your thigh muscles with stair step-ups, you take strain off your knees and hips. This is a particularly efficient exercise. **Level 2 or 3, page 65**

2. Lying Alternating Arm Raise

Down on the ground for this simple, wonderful exercise for your back (yes, it is the back muscle pulling your arm up!). **Level 1, page 90**

Program continues >

• Whenever you have music on, tap your toes or bounce your knee to the rhythm.

• Insist on bagging your own groceries at the food store.

Get two workouts in one. You can burn a substantial amount of extra calories during a strength workout if you move quickly from one exercise to the next. By keeping in motion rather than resting between exercises, you are combining strengthening with aerobic exercise, greatly boosting your energy burn. Key trick: Alternate between upper- and lower-body moves, so you give just-exercised muscles time to rest.

Track your metabolism. Even if you boost your metabolism, how would you know? It's largely been a matter of guesswork or cumulative results on the bathroom scale. Now, however, health providers and fitness centres can help clients track their resting metabolic rate (RMR)—the basic measure of metabolism—using a new device called the BodyGem. When you breathe into the handheld inhaler-like unit for a few minutes, your current RMR pops up on a digital readout, giving you a calorie goal for both diet and exercise—and a tangible way to check on your progress. To find healthcare professionals or gyms using the BodyGem, check a locator feature on the manufacturer's website, **www.healthetech.com**. ■

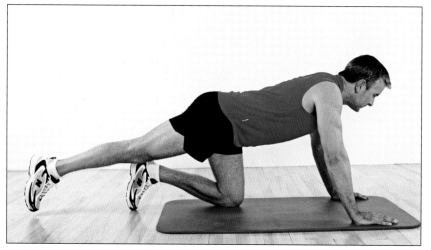

3. Lower-Body Extension

Another gentle yet effective strengthening move for your hips and back.
Level 1, page 90

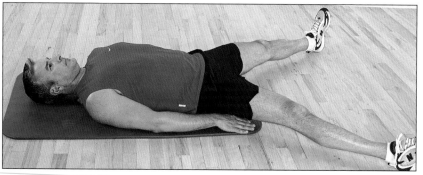

4. Lying Hip Abduction

Give yourself space and move slowly to do this terrific hip exercise
properly. **Level 1, page 61**

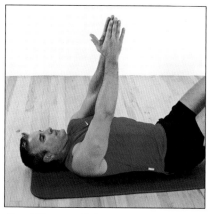

5. Chest Fly

You might be surprised how this
seemingly natural move gives your
chest muscles a good workout.
Level 1, page 96

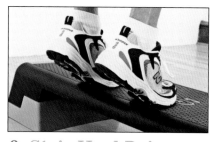

6. Stair Heel Raise

By doing this on a stair, you
lengthen the upward and downward movement, giving an even
better workout for your calves,
ankles and feet. **Level 2, page 104**

AEROBIC PROGRAM

Do your aerobic activity 4 to
6 days a week, progressing as
your comfort level allows, following these guidelines:

■ If you're new to cardiovascular exercise, begin by walking 2 minutes at a slow,
leisurely pace followed by 1 to
2 minutes of brisk walking.

■ Once you're comfortable
exercising for a total of 5 minutes, gradually boost the brisk
walking period by 30 to 60
seconds per week.

■ Build up gradually to a routine in which you walk at a
leisurely pace for 2 to 5 minutes, then walk briskly the rest
of the time. Build your total
walking time to between
20 and 40 minutes.

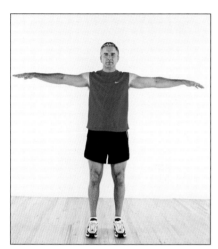

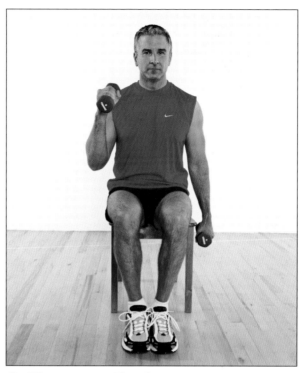

7. Around the World

Feel like a child again with these large but precise arm movements that aid your shoulders. **Level 2, page 78**

8. Hammer Curl

A slight twist on the standard biceps curl that offers a greater challenge to your largest arm muscle. **Level 2, page 111**

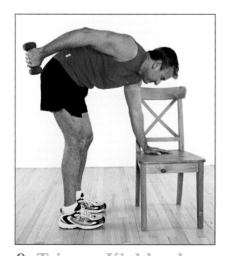

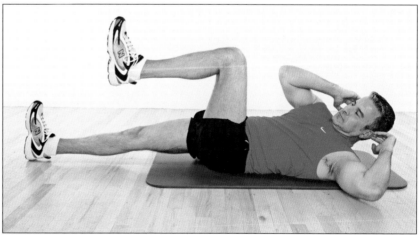

9. Triceps Kickback

Triceps are often much weaker than your biceps, so do this gently and carefully and don't push too hard at first. **Level 2, page 111**

10. Basic or Advanced Bicycle

Great for your abs, but also a wonderful calorie burner. **Level 2 or 3 depending on variation, page 83 or 85**

■ ADVANCED Strength Program

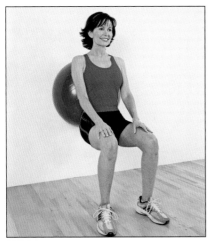

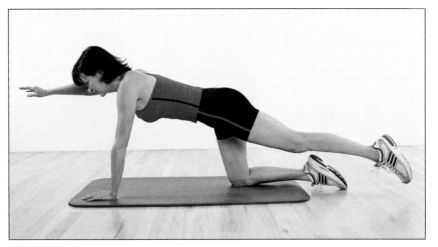

1. Ball Squat

A challenging first exercise that tests your thigh muscles and supports your knees and hips. **Level 3, page 67**

2. Bird Dog

Now onto your hands and knees for this leg-extending exercise that supports your hips and back. **Level 2, page 91**

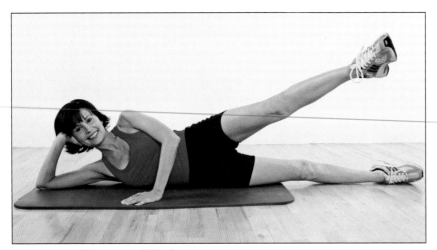

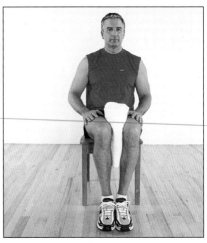

3. Side Thrust Kick

From hands and knees to your side for this interesting and challenging move for your hips. **Level 3, page 67**

4. Towel Squeeze

Back up into a chair for this simple isometric exercise for stronger leg muscles that again aid your hips. **Level 1, page 62**

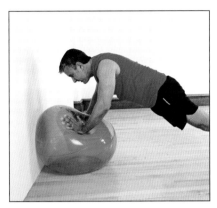

5. Ball Push-Up

Grab the exercise ball again and down on the floor for this challenging chest workout that also tests your balance. **Level 3, page 97**

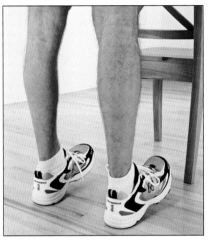

6. Heel/Toe Raise

Great for your feet and ankles, but also for your calf muscles. **Level 2, page 105**

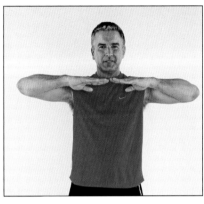

7. Upright Row

This shoulder exercise also forces a good-sized stretch of your elbow joint. **Level 2, page 77**

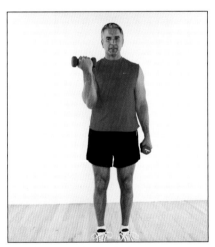

8. Standing Biceps Curl

This classic exercise is not only for good-looking arms but also elbow relief and extra calorie burn. **Level 3, page 112**

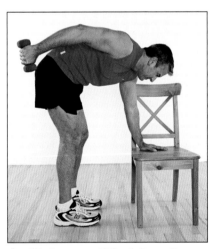

9. Triceps Kickback

Muscle pairs need balance and so for every biceps exercise you do, you need a triceps exercise. **Level 2, page 111**

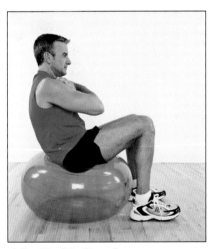

10. Ball Curl

One more time with your exercise ball. This exercise strengthens your abdominal muscles and truly tests your balance. **Level 3, page 85**

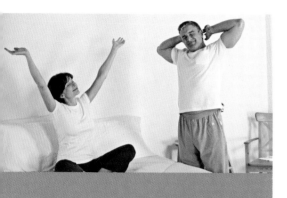

Aside from pain, the most devastating consequence of arthritis is its ability to rob you of movement and prevent you from going

about normal daily activities. These programs build strength and range of motion in all the body's major joints and muscle groups, but focus especially on large muscles that are important for gross motor functions such as walking, climbing stairs, lifting and doing household chores.

Instructions

Again, we have provided beginning, intermediate and advanced programs. For each program, there are two main sequences: strengthening and stretching. Here is how to proceed:

■ Do a five-minute warmup to get blood flowing throughout your body. Walking in place will do just fine.

■ Proceed with the strength exercises. Beginners should start with one set of 6 repetitions for each exercise; intermediate, one set of 6 to 8 repetitions; and advanced, one set of 8 repetitions.

■ Next, shift to the flexibility exercises.

■ BEGINNING Strength Program

making the
Program Work

Each of the three programs uses a different set of exercises and stretches. If you find some to be too easy or difficult, look at exercises prescribed for the same area of the body in the next level up or down. But if possible, try to follow the program as outlined. What to do when the workout gets too easy? Follow the progression guidelines outlined in the Total Body Stretch and Total Body Strength programs. Boiled down, they say to start with a low number of repetitions and build toward higher repetitions and multiple sets as you become stronger. These programs should take under 30 minutes.

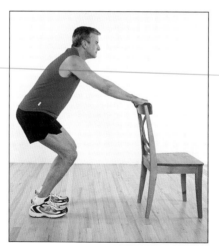

1. Partial Squat

Start your program by lengthening thigh muscles that support both hips and knees. **Level 1 or 2, page 61**

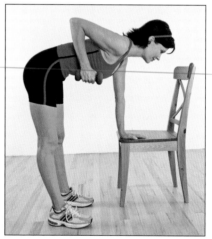

2. Bent Single Arm Row

This deceptively challenging exercise is for your back, not your arms! No weights makes it easier. **Level 1 or 2, page 92**

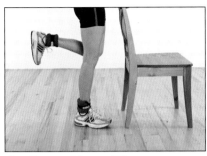

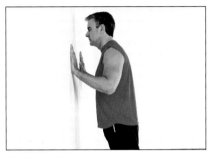

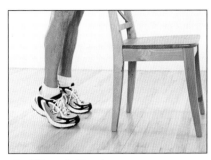

3. Standing Knee Flexion

A simple but effective exercise for your knees and hips. **Level 2, page 64**

4. Wall Push-Up

This modified version of the classic military exercise gently challenges your chest muscles. **Level 1, page 95**

5. Heel Raise

A simple but effective workout for your ankles and feet. Do it anywhere, anytime. **Level 1, page 104**

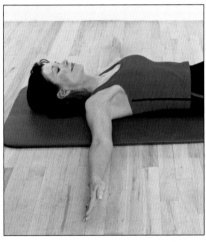

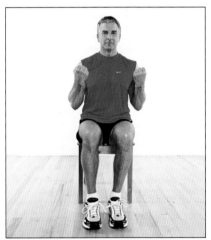

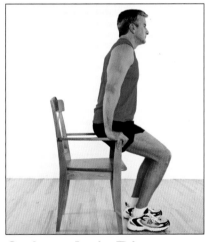

6. Lying Lateral Raise

Down on your back, slowly and carefully, to do this wonderful shoulder workout. **Level 1, page 75**

7. Seated Biceps Curl

Up into a chair so you can do this classic elbow-enhancing exercise. **Level 1, page 109**

8. Armchair Dip

Carefully lower and raise yourself for arm strength and elbow support. **Level 1, page 110**

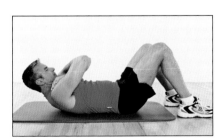

9. Basic or Advanced Abdominal Curl

End your strengthening sequence with this classic stomach test and turn the page for your flexibility routine! **Level 2 or 3, page 82 or 84**

■ BEGINNING Flexibility Program

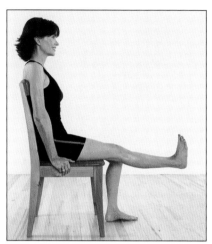

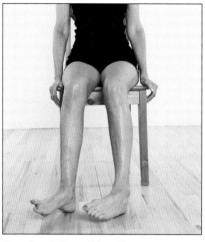

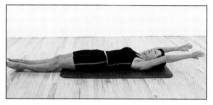

1. Seated Knee Extension

Gentle and easy, but hold it for best effect. Add weights to your ankle and you have a wonderful leg-strengthening exercise.
Page 56

2. Ankle Circle

Again, gentle and easy, but surprisingly refreshing for your feet. Walk around and you'll see. **Page 102**

3. Lying Total Body Stretch

The most natural of movements—you see wild animals do it all the time—and for good reason: it refreshes and rejuvenates. **Page 81**

everyday
secrets

THE GROCERIES

Sometimes hard on joints but also hard to avoid, grocery shopping—with its reaching, grasping, lifting, hauling, loading and putting away—can be a challenging chore when you have arthritis. To make the job easier:

Bolster your bags. Why struggle wrestling groceries in paper bags without handles or plastic bags that pinch your hands under heavy loads? Alternative: Bring your own cloth bags with thick handles made of canvas or wooden dowels (sometimes provided by libraries, offered as premiums from charities such as public broadcasting or available from retailers such as Mountain Equipment Co-op). Tell the checkout clerk how heavy you want the bags: When the weight is comfortable for your hands, carrying will work the muscles of your shoulders, arms and back. Start with light loads and add an extra item each time you go shopping.

Walk the aisles. Don't aimlessly wander the grocery aisles—purposely make it a goal to stroll down every one of them, whether you need to pick something off the shelves or not. You'll build extra steps of walking into your day and may actually remember to pick up the paprika you ran out of last week. If browsing along the way makes it too tempting to pick up food you don't need, stick to the perimeter of the store (where healthy foods like fresh produce tend to be) or circulate through aisles you've already shopped.

Unload piecemeal. When you get home with your groceries, avoid loading yourself down with multiple bags. Instead, get one bag from the car at a time, which prevents pain from stressing arthritic joints while building strength and adding to your daily accumulation of steps.

Bag it yourself. First, the exercise is good for you. Second, you can organize your bags for easier unloading when at home. And third, you'll win friends by helping speed up the checkout line, since fewer and fewer grocery stores have baggers. ■

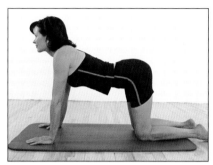

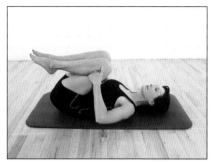

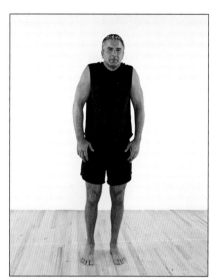

4. Cat Stretch

A little more strenuous, but again, very natural and wonderful for your back. **Page 88**

5. Knees to Chest

Chances are you spent many hours of your childhood in this position. Stretch your back again and regain your youthful spirit. **Page 59**

6. Shoulder Roll

When your neck or upper back aches, you do this move naturally for relief. Do it now for flexibility and shoulder relief. **Page 72**

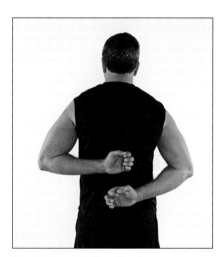

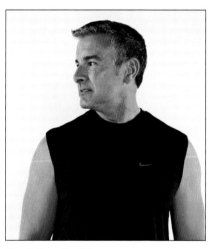

7. Knuckle Rub

At first, this seems difficult. But in time, you will find your knuckles will rise farther up your back as your body grows more flexible. **Page 73**

8. Neck Turn

End this routine with yet another movement we do naturally to relieve tension and provide soothing relief. **Page 98**

5 Greater Mobility

■ INTERMEDIATE Strength Program

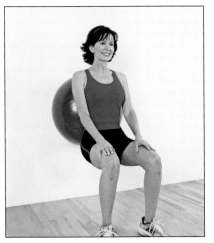

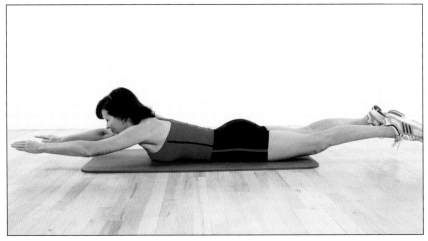

1. Ball Squat

This is challenging in two ways: Squats truly test your leg muscles and balancing the large ball takes practice. But the benefits are great! **Level 3, page 67**

2. Superman

You'd think this would be an arm and leg exercise, but it is the muscles in your torso that provide the lift and balance. **Level 2, page 91**

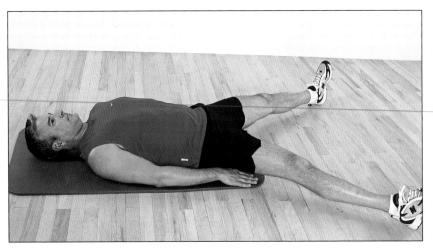

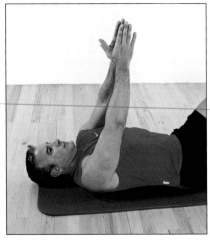

3. Lying Hip Abduction

No need to try doing a full split! Gently open your legs until you feel tension and stop. In time, you will be able to widen the split. **Level 1, page 61**

4. Chest Fly

This seems natural and easy, but the weight of your arms makes for a surprisingly good workout. **Level 1, page 96**

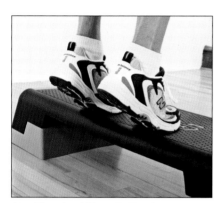

5. Stair Heel Raise

While you will feel the muscle tension in your calf muscles, this is a very beneficial exercise for your ankles and feet. **Level 2, page 104**

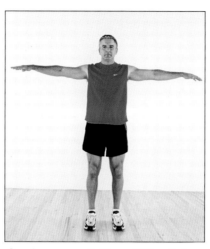

6. Around the World

Next, this shoulder exercise will help you reach more assuredly for things above your head. **Level 2, page 78**

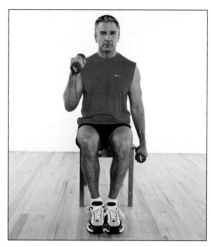

7. Hammer Curl

This variation of the classic biceps curl will provide much relief to your elbow joint. **Level 2, page 111**

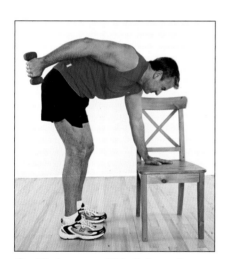

8. Triceps Kickback

Be prepared to feel the tension and fatigue in this upper-arm muscle, which often goes unexercised. **Level 2, page 111**

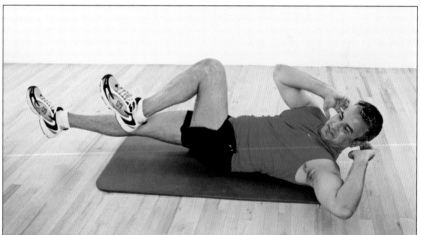

9. Basic or Advanced Bicycle

Great for your abdomen, great for your legs and even great for your heart and lungs. **Level 2 or 3 depending on variation, page 83 or 85**

■ INTERMEDIATE Flexibility Program

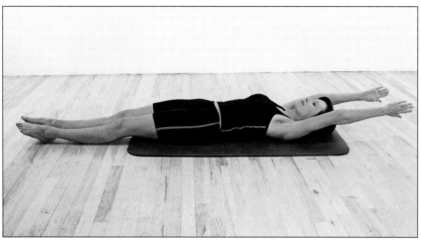

1. Lying Total Body Stretch

We recommend this stretch often because it feels so good, so natural and so relieving. **Page 94**

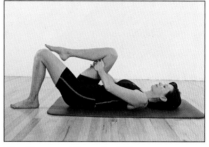

2. Low Back Knees to Chest

Don't worry if at first you have a hard time with this move. In time, you'll feel comfortable on your back and with your knees pulled to you. **Page 86**

everyday *secrets*

YOUR DAILY DOINGS

As you move throughout your day, you'll benefit from knowing a number of basic skills or tools such as these:

Practice perfect lifts. Doing your workout isn't the only time good form is important. Household tasks are exercise too—and it's just as important to perform everyday movements properly to keep from straining joints and muscles. Lifting objects such as laundry baskets or stacks of newspapers can be particularly hard on the back. But done correctly, lifting can also provide a good workout for muscles and joints. Here's how:

• Get close to the object and try to keep it near your centre of gravity, which makes it easier to lift and is less likely to strain your back.

• Keep your back straight and bend at the knees to raise the object off the ground. Avoid bending at the waist and trying to muscle something up using just your back. (If you have knee problems, don't be afraid to ask for help.)

• Once you've completed the lift, don't turn at the waist, but keep the object close to your body, point your toes where you want to go and turn your entire body.

Stand without strain. When standing for prolonged periods (for example, at the kitchen counter washing dishes or preparing food), take pressure off the lower back by resting one foot on a platform

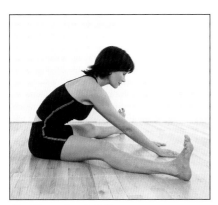

3. Seated V

Another great stretch that seems awkward at first, but becomes natural with just a little practice. **Page 57**

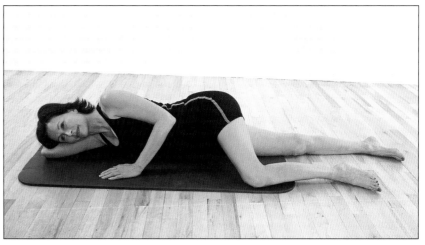

4. Lying Pelvis Rotation

While still on the ground, get on your side and do this gentle stretch for the muscles along the outside of the thigh. **Page 59**

Program continues >

about two to four inches high—about the height of a phone book—and occasionally shifting weight from one foot to another. To fight fatigue while standing, do what you'd think would make you more tired: Exercise. Heel raises squeeze your veins, prevent blood from pooling in your extremities and force blood back to your heart, which actually makes it less tiring to stand for a long time.

Take care on stairs. Going up and down stairs can be a major ordeal for people with arthritis, but going about it the right way can minimize pain or help prevent it from getting worse. Some ways to do it:

• Although the first priority is to do what's most comfortable, avoid taking steps one foot at a time, leading with the better foot. Constantly favouring one foot generally causes one side to become stronger than the other, making problems worse, not better. A better way: If it's safe to do so, take steps evenly using both feet, using the rail for support.

• Use your arms for support and balance, but don't use them to lift yourself up the stairs, which can lead to pain in the shoulders.

• Be particularly dedicated to exercises for the quadriceps muscles of the thighs, which are primary movers both for going up stairs and the more difficult braking action of going down.

Use a cane. Some people with arthritis feel using a cane makes them seem old or crippled, but it's

continued on page 158

5 Greater Mobility ■ ADVANCED

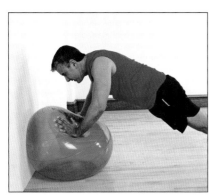

5. Ball Push-Up

This exercise is great for hands, arms, chest and overall balance and strength. **Level 3, page 97**

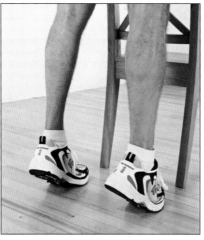

6. Heel/Toe Raise

While it is the calf muscles that get tested the most, this exercise is great for all parts of your feet. **Level 2, page 105**

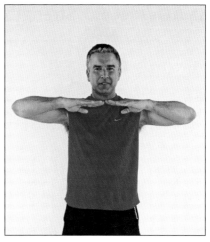

7. Upright Row

Strong chest muscles make all your lifting and throwing much, much easier to do. **Level 2, page 77**

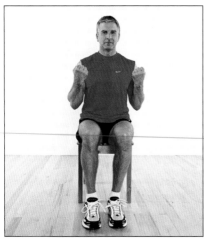

8. Seated Biceps Curl

Strong biceps will make lifting and carrying things much easier as well. **Level 2, page 109**

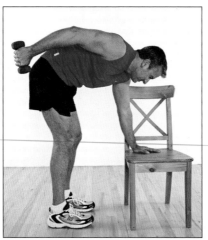

9. Triceps Kickback

Muscle pairs, like the biceps and triceps, need to be balanced, so don't neglect the less showy muscle opposite your biceps. **Level 2, page 111**

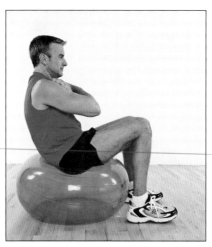

10. Ball Curl

End this mobility-strength program with an abdomen exercise that has a sense of fun and excitement. Don't fall off the ball! **Level 3, page 85**

■ ADVANCED Flexibility Program

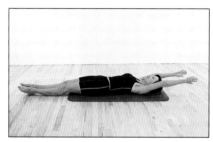

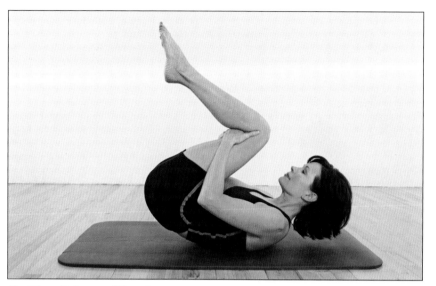

1. Lying Total Body Stretch

For optimal mobility, you want your entire body to be loose and flexible. This opening stretch gets you on your way. **Page 94**

2. Rocking Chair

At first, it might feel awkward to curl up on your back like this. But this stretch is soothing and effective. Do it on a carpet or mat for comfort. **Page 87**

Program continues >

---

everyday **secrets**

WORKING OUTSIDE

Just about any chore outdoors involves major joints and muscles important for mobility—which can make yard and garden tasks especially challenging. But the physical labour is good for your muscles, so it's worth doing all you can, with steps like the following to ease discomfort.

Fashion hefty handles. When using lawn and garden tools such as rakes and hoes, make the handles easier to grasp the way hockey players wearing mitts do: Wrap the handle in athletic tape to make it thicker—and wear gloves when working to protect sensitive hands.

Don't work too hard in the yard. Take a break every 15 minutes when gardening. It's easy to become engrossed in yard work, but while the labour counts as exercise, you want to avoid getting too much of a good thing, lest you overwork your abdomen and lower back. Frequent rests help your muscles relax and make the work more pleasant. In addition, switch sides frequently to avoid overworking a single muscle group—and use exercises such as the bicycle to get your torso into shape.

continued on page 162

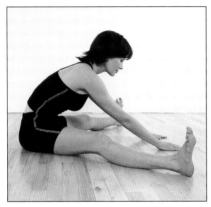

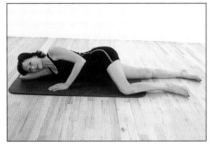

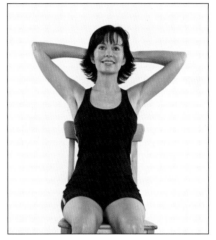

3. Seated V

Now into a seated position with legs straight out. This stretch is great for your hips and challenges your whole body. **Page 57**

4. Lying Pelvis Rotation

Lie down on your back and get those legs rolling above you. Outstanding for your hips and a general feel-good move as well. **Page 59**

5. Seated Chest Stretch

Back up to a chair—or even standing, if you like—to stretch the often-tense muscles at the top of your chest and the front of your shoulders. **Page 94**

continued from page 161

Give yourself a raise. Planting a garden doesn't have to take place at ground level. Instead of stooping to the dirt, use raised beds so you can exercise your green thumb from a seated or standing position.

Take a seat. Kneeling for planting or weeding can be hard on knees. A better position: Sitting low to the ground on a bucket, stool or small wagon. Check gardening centres, catalogues or websites for garden carts that can be loaded and pulled, but close with a lid that doubles as a seat. Alternative position: Try lying on your hip or side for tasks such as hand digging or weeding.

Cushion your knees. If you need to kneel and your joints comfortably allow it, use pads made of closed-cell foam, which cushions without compressing flat. You can order knee pads and other tools for the garden from Internet websites such as **rittenhouse.ca**.

Take the rigour from raking. When raking, use short strokes instead of reaching away from the body, which puts more stress on joints and the back. Bend your knees slightly when stroking, to allow muscles of the legs and hips to contribute more to the motion. Plus, this posture eases strain on the upper body and protects your back.

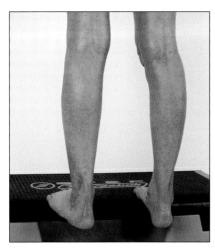

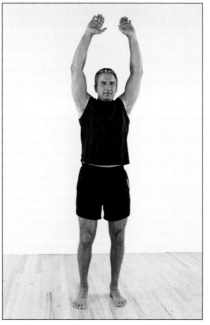

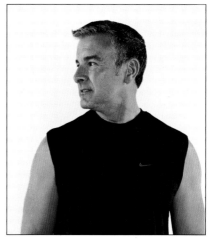

6. Stair Calf Stretch

Chances are you'll "feel the burn" in your calves as you do this classic stretch for your lower legs and ankles. **Page 102**

7. 'Good Morning' Exercise

Wonderful for your shoulders. Feel your rib cage spread and take in some deep breaths to refresh your whole body. **Page 74**

8. Neck Turn

The classic way to end a stretching routine. Tension often lands in your neck, so let it release. **Page 98**

Throw in the trowel. Digging with a trowel can be tough on arthritic hands. To make it easier, start with the narrowest implement you can find: Tools with wider blades create more resistance in the dirt. When digging, chop with the trowel to loosen clumped dirt, then insert the trowel no deeper than half its length to loosen the soil and avoid straining against more densely packed deeper layers. Work your way deeper with short scoops.

Be sure with a shovel. As with a trowel, you want to dig with a shovel in shallow bits, gradually loosening dirt in small shovelfuls. Use your legs to lift the dirt, doing a partial squat to gain leverage, keeping hands close to your body to avoid stressing your back. Avoid placing the shovel too far in front of you. Instead, keep the load within a couple of feet (about a half-metre) to promote better posture and balance as you work. If you place the shovel farther than that, lunge forward with one knee to keep your body's centre of gravity close to the load.

Work standing up. When planting seeds, sharpen one end of a broomstick to make holes in the soil, then drop seeds from a standing position using a long piece of small-diameter PVC piping cut to about waist height. ■

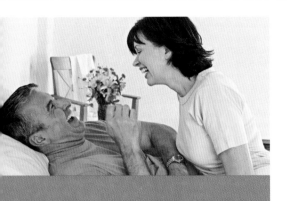

Dexterity usually refers to fine motor control—the ability to write, draw, cook, pick up objects with your fingers and work with tools

or crafts. But you need more than nimble fingers to use hands effectively; you also need strong and supple muscles in the upper body, especially around the shoulders, upper back, front of the chest and arms. Stabilizing this area, known as the shoulder girdle, provides greater control, endurance and overall function of your extremities, allowing more refined movements in the hands and wrists.

Instructions

We've provided beginning, intermediate and advanced programs. For each program, there are two main sequences: strengthening and stretching. Here is how to proceed:

■ Do a five-minute warmup to get blood flowing throughout your body. Walking in place will do just fine, though since this is an upper-body program, be sure your arms have participated in the warmup.

■ Proceed with the strength exercises. Beginners should start with one set of 6 repetitions for each exercise; intermediate, one set of 6 to 8 repetitions; and advanced, one set of 8 repetitions.

■ Next, shift to the flexibility exercises.

making the
Program Work

These programs consist entirely of upper-body exercises and stretches. Progress in the order indicated, starting with large muscles that support the extremities and working toward finer movements of the hands and wrists. Follow the progression guidelines outlined in the Total Body Stretch and Total Body Strength programs, beginning strength programs with the starting number of sets and repetitions indicated.

■ BEGINNING Strength Program

Starting point: 1 set of 6 repetitions

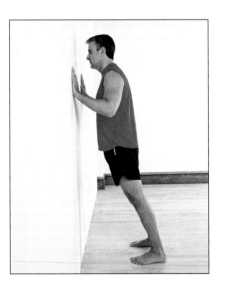

1. Wall Push-Up

This standing version of the classic floor push-up still gives your chest and arms a good workout. **Level 1, page 95**

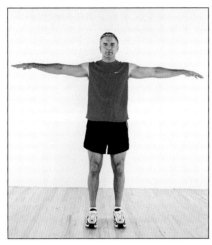

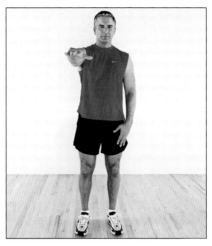

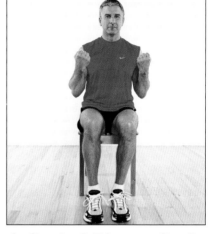

2. Standing Lateral Raise

Use the weight of your arms to build up shoulder and neck muscles. **Level 2, page 77**

3. Front Raise

Similar to lateral raises, but this exercise strengthens a different set of shoulder and back muscles. **Level 2, page 78**

4. Seated Biceps Curl

You may not think that strong upper arms will help your dexterity, but they offer key support to your elbows and shoulders. **Level 1, page 109**

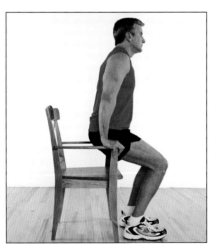

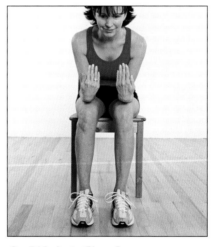

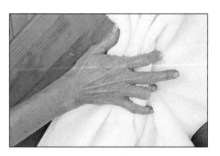

5. Armchair Dip

While the main muscles strengthened here are in your arms, this everyday movement is great for overall dexterity and motion. **Level 1, page 110**

6. Wrist Curl

Now to the muscles of the wrist and forearm. Though smaller in size than the upper-arm muscles, they need strengthening too. **Level 1, page 116**

7. Towel Grab

End this routine with a simple exercise for stronger fingers and hands. **All levels, page 121**

6 Greater Dexterity BEGINNING ■ INTERMEDIATE

■ BEGINNING Flexibility Program

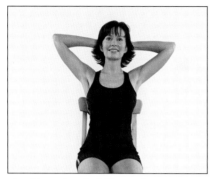

1. Seated Chest Stretch

Use the weight of your arms to provide your chest muscles a long, full stretch. **Page 94**

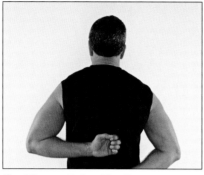

2. Knuckle Rub

Now stretch your upper arms and shoulder joint by carefully gliding your knuckles along your spine. **Page 73**

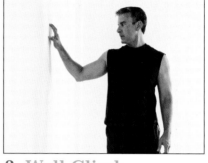

3. Wall Climb

Don't be self-conscious doing this stretch and don't rush through it. It is particularly good for people with limited dexterity. **Page 73**

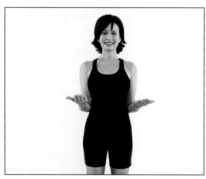

4. Forearm Flip

This both stretches and strengthens the muscles in your forearm, making elbow and wrist movement easier. **Page 108**

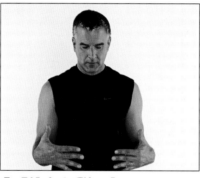

5. Wrist Circle

A relatively small movement, but wrist stretches like these can make all the difference in your everyday functioning. **Page 115**

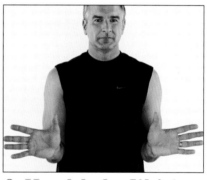

6. Handshake Wrist Bend

Another wrist stretch that uses a different motion to help your manual dexterity. **Page 114**

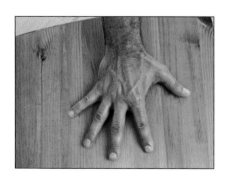

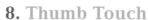

7. Finger Stretch

Don't think that because you use fingers all day, they don't need strengthening and stretching. This flex does wonders! **Page 120**

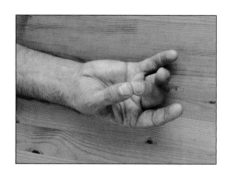

8. Thumb Touch

Finally, end your dexterity workout with this simple sequence for your hands and fingers. **Page 120**

■ INTERMEDIATE Strength Program

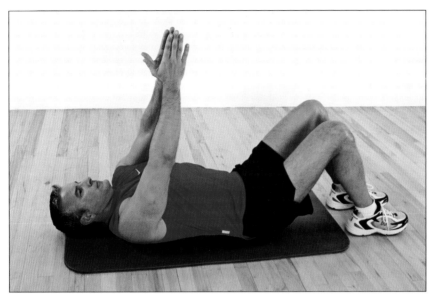

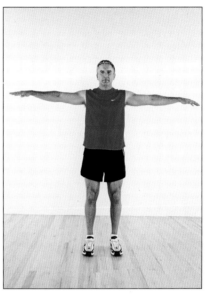

1. Chest Fly

Lying on your back, you are strengthening your chest, arms and shoulders with this unweighted arm lift. **Level 1, page 96**

2. Around the World

Now back on your feet to move your arms from another perspective, giving them a full range of motion as well as more strength. **Level 2, page 78**

Program continues >

---

everyday *secrets*

CLOTHING

When fingers and wrists ache, when bending and pulling are a challenge, getting dressed can become an ordeal. While exercises and stretches can improve your ability to dress easily, you can also take steps to make the routine easier:

Buy big. Instead of buying clothes—especially shirts, blouses, jackets and sweatshirts—with perfect fit in mind, choose items that

are a size too big through the body or made with a roomy cut, to give you extra room when wrestling them on and off. Avoid items that lack "give," such as denim and tweed or are difficult to get over your head, such as turtlenecks.

Cut demands on hands. Choose pants with elastic waists that are easy to pull on and off, sparing your hands painful manipulation of buttons or zippers. When you can't avoid the use of fasteners, choose items such as skirts, dresses, shirts, blouses and bras

that zip or fasten on the side or front instead the back. If you're stuck with difficult-to-reach fasteners, try positioning the garment so you can reach a zipper, button or clasp in front, then move the item into proper position. When possible, use fasteners made with Velcro or large, flat buttons that are easy to handle.

Reorganize your closet. An organized closet doesn't just look better—it might make you feel better. Instead of heaping shoes

continued on page 168

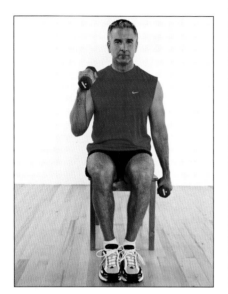

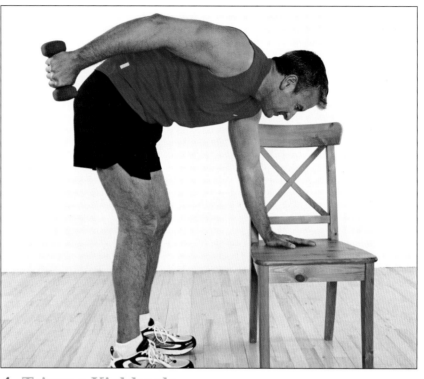

3. Hammer Curl

This seated curl strengthens forearm muscles that help support your elbow, working on a different part of the arm from biceps curls. **Level 2, page 111**

4. Triceps Kickback

Use an armless chair or a bench for this exercise that works on the muscles at the bottom of your upper arm. **Level 2, page 111**

continued from page 167

on the floor of your closet—where you have to bend and sort them—get a hanging shoe rack for a wall or door so footwear is within easy reach. And if reaching for hangers at or above shoulder height is difficult, lower the bar of your hanging rack. Meantime, take items off the rack using two hands or grasping items between a hand and your arm or wrist.

Prepare for morning. If you know you're going to feel stiff in the morning, lay out clothes the night

before, when it's easier to search through closets, paw through drawers and handle the items you choose.

Be deliberate with drawers. Most dressers come with bottom drawers that are larger and tough to open. Though it's natural to organize drawers by content size, with bulky things in bigger drawers, think instead in terms of how often clothes are used, putting frequently worn items in smaller drawers closer to the top, where they're easier to reach and handle.

Sit to stand. To make putting on pants easier (and to make sure pain while dressing doesn't cause you to lose your balance), sit down on the edge of a bed or chair to pull trousers over your legs, then stand up to hitch the waist.

Do the splits. They're popular with kids, but immensely useful for people with arthritis—pants with zippers in the legs that can turn a pair of long trousers into shorts without taking the entire garment off and replacing it with another. You can get them at stores catering to young shoppers, but a better bet

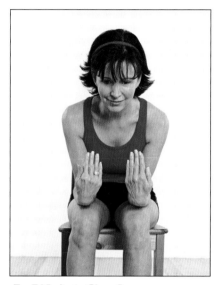

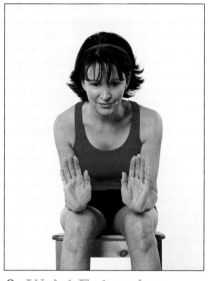

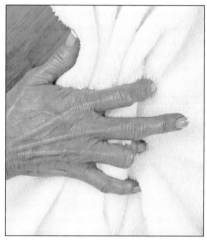

5. Wrist Curl

Back in a chair, you can now start toning up muscles closer to your hands—those of your wrists—that support your hands as they tackle jobs like piano playing or sewing.
Level 1, page 116

6. Wrist Extension

Here you are working on the muscles opposite the ones you put to use in the wrist curls, a balance that helps both sets of muscles.
Level 1, page 116

7. Towel Grab

A seemingly silly exercise that a pet cat might think was a game for its pleasure is designed to help rebuild dexterity in stiff fingers.
All levels, page 121

may be sporting goods stores or catalogues, which often feature lightweight convertible clothes for hiking and multi-sport activities.

Use donning devices. You'll find it easier to get into a variety of garments with special devices designed to help with manipulation. (Check a medical supply store or Internet websites such as **aidsforarthritis.com** or **independent-needs.com)** Devices include:

• buttonhooks, featuring a handle holding a wire that grasps buttons and pulls them through buttonholes

• sock aids, in which a shell holds the sock in place as you slip your foot into it and allows you to pull it up using long handles

• long shoehorns with extended handles that allow you to get feet into shoes without bending over

• zipper pullers, which grab zippers with a hook and allow you to slide them with the help of a handle

Focus on footwear. Getting shoes on is half the battle. The other half is getting them to stay. Laces can be hard on arthritic fingers, but if they're made of elastic, you

need only tie shoes once and they'll stay snapped tight until you want your shoes off. Some stylish shoes now on the market come already laced with knot-free elastic cord: You just slip the shoes on and off without tying anything—the elastic conforms to your foot. Other options include shoes that close with Velcro. ■

5 Greater Dexterity ■ INTERMEDIATE

■ **INTERMEDIATE** Flexibility Program

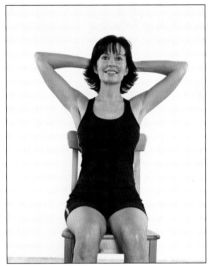

1. Seated Chest Stretch

You can sit or stand while you try to lengthen the muscles of your upper chest and the front of your shoulders; as you repeat, your arms will go further back. **Page 94**

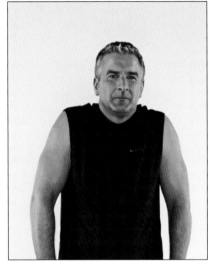

2. Shoulder Roll

A good stretch for your shoulders, this is also a relaxing exercise for tense shoulder and neck muscles. **Page 72**

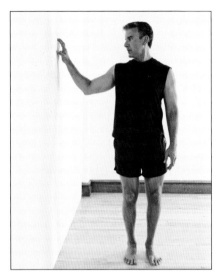

3. Wall Climb

Working out both your shoulders and your fingers, this exercise helps increase your shoulder muscles' range of motion. **Page 73**

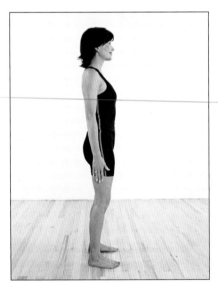

4. Arm Hang

For elbows that are stiff and bent, this stretch helps you gradually straighten your arm all the way again. **Page 108**

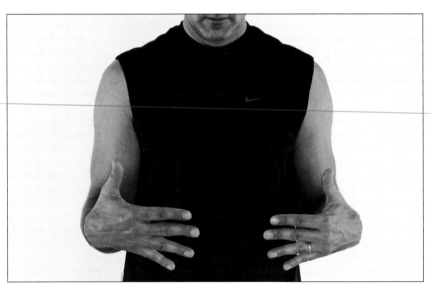

5. Wrist Circle

This simple stretch, which seems like drawing circles in the air, incorporates all the movements of the wrist in a continuous motion. **Page 115**

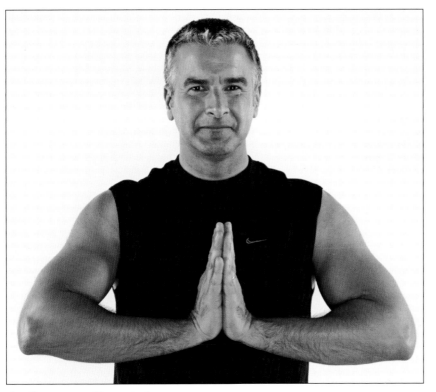

6. Prayer Stretch

This pious-looking stretch lengthens muscles in your elbows, forearms and wrists. **Page 115**

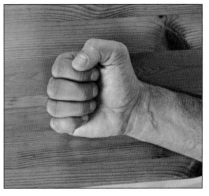

7. Gentle Fist

The movements of this stretch give your fingers a relaxing work-out while also expanding their range of motion. **Page 120**

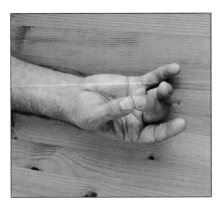

8. Thumb Touch

Finger dexterity depends on the movements of this stretch, which involves each finger individually. And remember: You can do this anytime! **Page 120**

6 Greater Dexterity ■ ADVANCED

■ **ADVANCED** Strength Program Starting point: 1 set of 8 repetitions.

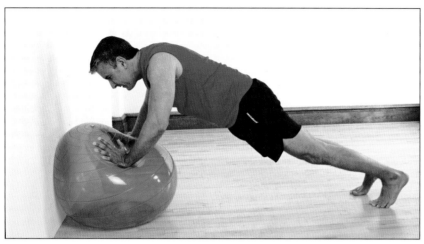

1. Ball Push-Up

Now you're working out the larger muscles that support your arms and hands in a strength exercise that also requires balance. **Level 3, page 97**

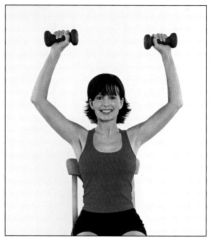

2. Overhead Dumbbell Press

On to an armless chair or bench for this classic exercise that strengthens your shoulders, upper back and upper arms. **Level 3, page 79**

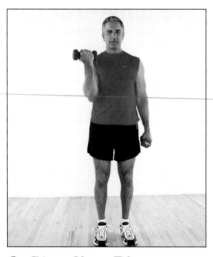

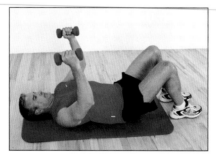

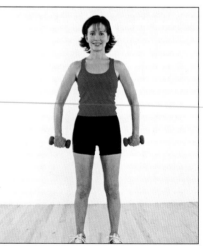

3. Standing Biceps Curl

Stand up for this set of curls—it works muscles in your torso and lower body as well as your shoulder and arms because it requires some balance. **Level 3, page 112**

4. Lying Triceps Extension

Back on the mat for more shoulder and arm work, giving a strong base to your wrists and hands. **Level 3, page 113**

5. Standing Wrist Curl

There is a twist to these curls that affects muscles in your forearms not touched by other curls. **Level 3, page 119**

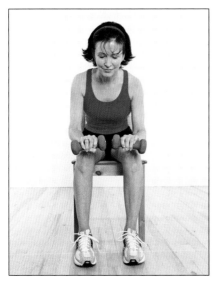

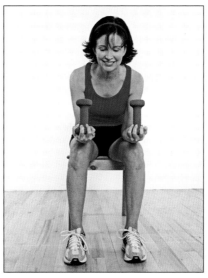

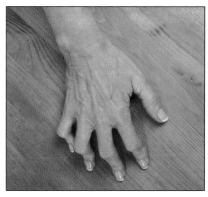

6. Weighted Wrist Extension

Sit down for this exercise, which strengthens the muscles of your wrists with repetition, then greater weights. **Level 2, page 118**

7. Thor's Hammer

Still in your chair, grab the weights by their ends for this rotation exercise that also strengthens your wrists. **Level 3, page 119**

8. Spider Walk

Fingers are the beneficiaries of this tabletop exercise that can be done with all fingers at once or with individual ones as you get stronger. **All levels, page 121**

everyday *secrets*

IN THE KITCHEN

Cooking is not only a necessity but, for many of us, a pleasure. Here are ways to make the process easier when arthritis challenges your dexterity:

Leverage lids. You can use an electric can opener to take the tops off most cans, but pop-top cans for products such as soft drinks, pet food, nuts or canned cake icing often lack the metal lip that an opener requires to work. Options: Use a knife to pry the top off a pop can or use the handle of a spoon as a lever to take off a vacuum pack lid. Otherwise, try flipping the can over: The bottom may be the right shape for your can opener. To loosen tight lids on small bottles, reach for a nutcracker: The toothy, gripping gap for the nut is the perfect size for grasping and wrenching bottle caps.

Strain, don't drain. Instead of hefting a pot of boiled food to the sink so you can dump water through a strainer, get a pot with a perforated insert that holds food but can be lifted out of the water, leaving the heavy pot behind. Have a family member on cleanup duty dump the water later.

Choose the right knife. Cutting with a regular knife may prove difficult when arthritis affects

continued on page 174

6 Greater Dexterity

■ ADVANCED Flexibility Program

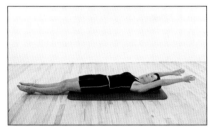

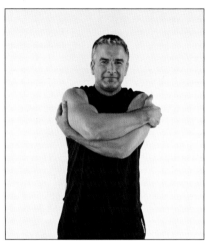

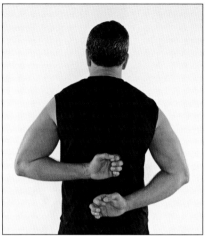

1. Total Body Stretch

Standing or lying in bed, this great stretch gets the kinks out and makes your whole body feel better. **Page 94**

2. Self-Hug

You're not just building self-esteem with this hug; you're stretching muscles in the back of your shoulders. **Page 72**

3. Knuckle Rub

The more you practice this behind-your-back stretch, the farther up your spine you'll be able to go as you stretch the muscles of your shoulders and upper arms. **Page 73**

continued from page 173

hands and wrists, but special L-shaped knives allow you to grip an upright handle that keeps stress off your wrist. In some cases, you can also make what you're cutting easier to deal with: Soaking potatoes in warm water, for example, softens the skin and makes them less challenging to peel.

Arrange for reaching. No kitchen seems to have enough cabinet space, but to make best use of yours, use the lower cupboards for the items you use most frequently, to cut down on the need to reach over your head, putting stress on your shoulder joints. Next priority: Put heavier items on lower shelves and lighter ones up higher. If you find you need to reach overhead often, try using a tool that features a pincher grip on the end of a long handle that can be used to pick up a variety of objects.

Take cups from cupboards. To clear room from cabinets so you can manage their contents more effectively, take frequently used cups out of the cupboard altogether and instead hang them from pegs underneath.

Jump-start juicing. Save yourself effort when using a hand juicer for oranges or grapefruits by rolling the fruit firmly on the counter with your palm before you slice and juice. The pressure will loosen the flesh from the rind and boost your juice output. ■

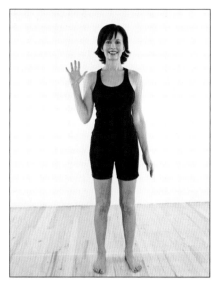

4. Shoulder Touch

Your arms go to your sides for this elbow-bending stretch; keep your elbows close to your waist throughout. **Page 109**

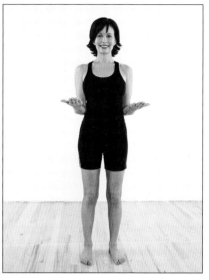

5. Forearm Flip

Here's another elbow stretch that works on range of motion in that often-stiff joint. **Page 108**

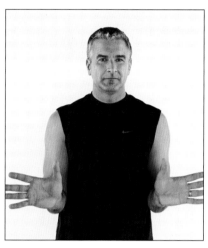

6. Handshake Wrist Bend

Keep your hands moving in this stretch designed primarily for the wrists. **Page 114**

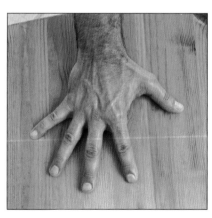

7. Finger Stretch

Separate your fingers as far as you can; then relax and do it again. It will feel great. **Page 120**

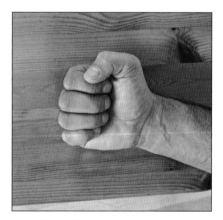

8. Gentle Fist

Slowly curling up and opening stiff joints will help them become more nimble again. **Page 120**

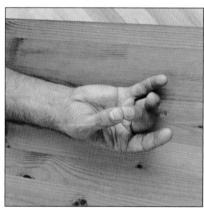

9. Thumb Touch

Here's a good way to check on the mobility of all your fingers and keep them moving at the same time. **Page 120**

7 Golf

Those who play regularly know that golf is a pleasure that is hard to give up. If arthritis is hampering your game, try to make this diverse program of exercise and stretches a three-times-a-week habit. A golf swing is a total body activity that gets much of its power from the lower body and back. The twisting and rotation of each stroke can be hard even on people without arthritis, so you'll need to strengthen and improve mobility of joints and muscles involved with multiple planes of motion, particularly in the hips and spine.

■ Strength Exercises

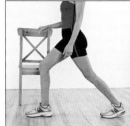
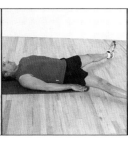
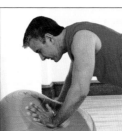
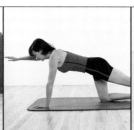
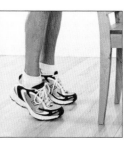

1. Partial Stationary Lunge
Level 3, page 68

2. Lying Hip Abduction
Level 1, page 61

3. Ball Push-Up
Level 3, page 97

4. Bird Dog
Level 2, page 66

5. Heel Raise
Level 1, page 104

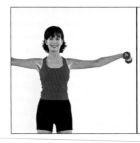
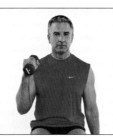
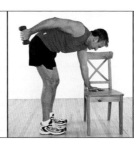
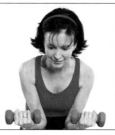
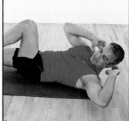

6. Weighted Lateral Raise
Level 3, page 79

7. Hammer Curl
Level 2, page 111

8. Triceps Kickback
Level 2, page 111

9. Weighted Wrist Curl
Level 2, page 117

10. Basic or Advanced Bicycle
Level 2 or 3 depending on variation, pages 83 or 85

Instructions

At least three times a week, get a 20-minute cardio-vascular workout, such as brisk walking or cycling. And at least twice a week, do this program of 10 strengthening exercises and 10 stretches. It seems like a lot, but can be finished in just 20 minutes. Try to do the exercises and stretches in the order given; they progress from large-muscle groups to small and rotate through different body areas so as not to overly test a single muscle group.

■ Flexibility Exercises

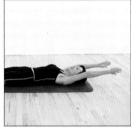

1. Lying Total Body Stretch
Page 94

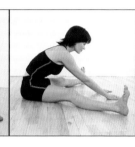

2. Rocking Chair
Page 87

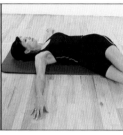

3. Seated V
Page 57

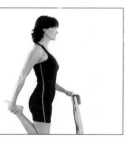

4. Pelvic Twist
Page 87

5. Standing Quad Stretch
Page 58

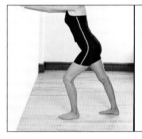

6. Runner's Calf Stretch
Page 103

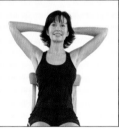

7. Seated Chest Stretch
Page 94

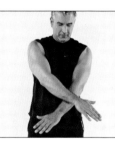

8. Scissors
Page 74

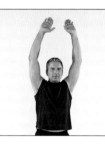

9. 'Good Morning' Exercise
Page 74

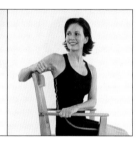

10. Seated Torso Twist
Page 80

make them easier to access. Try not to keep these things in your pocket, but rather strategically set yourself up, using your bag or your cart for easier access. For example, use a golf glove that has a snap-in ball marker.

Careful with the bending. In golf you are constantly picking up or putting down your ball. It's challenging for your back, neck and knees. If reaching to the ground over and over proves challenging, squat rather than bend at the waist.

Focus on the abs. When bolstering the torso, don't ignore the abdominal muscles, which support the spine and help power the torso: They're among the most neglected muscles among golfers—perhaps one reason the gut is one of the top areas for golf injuries, even among the pros. ■

9 Racket Sports

Tennis is a game you just never want to give up. But it is a tough sport on your body (The proof: How many top pros are competitive after the age of 35? Compare that to golf or baseball!) Tennis has many intense physical demands: pivoting, starting and stopping, moving quickly in all directions, swinging from all angles. There's not a joint in your body that racket sports don't test. For that reason, people with arthritis who stay with the game need to have a rigorous program to keep them healthy, fluid and having fun.

■ Strength Exercises

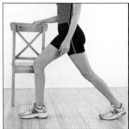

1. Partial Stationary Lunge
Level 3, page 68

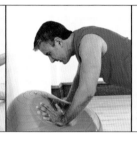

2. Side Thrust Kick
Level 3, page 67

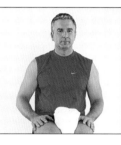

3. Ball Push-Up
Level 3, page 97

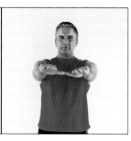

4. Towel Squeeze
Level 1, page 62

5. Around the World
Level 2, page 78

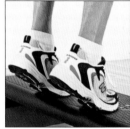

6. Stair Heel Raise
Level 2, page 104

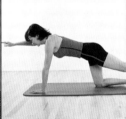

7. Bird Dog
Level 2, page 66

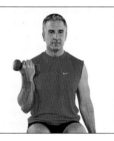

8. Biceps Curl
Level 2, page 110

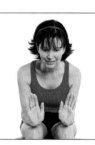

9. Wrist Extension
Level 1, page 116

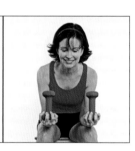

10. Thor's Hammer
Level 2, page 119

everyday *secrets*

ON THE COURT

Warm up before starting. Be sure to get your blood flowing and your joints and muscles loosened before starting a game. If not, you greatly increase your chances of joint pain and even injury.

Cushion the impact. It's essential to invest in a good pair of tennis shoes with superior padding to absorb the impact of body weight. Replace your shoes as soon as the heels begin to show wear, because they will no longer be giving you the support you need.

Feet of clay. Clay or Har-Tru courts are much kinder to your joints than hard courts. If you have the choice, always pick clay courts, where the surface absorbs the impact of your steps and you

Instructions

We suggest this three-part workout—aerobic, strengthening, then stretching—three times a week. For the aerobic component, do 20 to 30 minutes of brisk walking. As you become more fit, try to include short bouts (at least 15 seconds at a time) of jogging between 45-second periods of walking, to condition your body to the sport's constant changes of pace. Then do the 10 strength and 10 stretching moves listed here, which should take under 30 minutes. Start the strength exercises with one set of six repetitions. Hold your stretches at least 15 seconds.

■ Flexibility Exercises

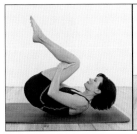 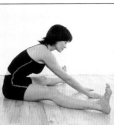 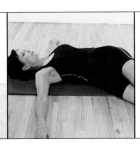 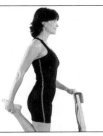 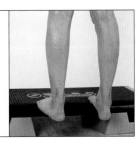

1. Rocking Chair
Page 87

2. Seated V
Page 57

3. Pelvic Twist
Page 87

4. Standing Quad Stretch
Page 58

5. Stair Calf Stretch
Page 102

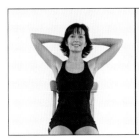 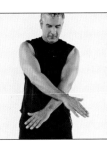 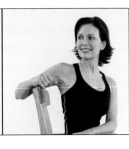 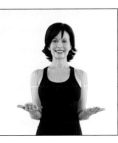 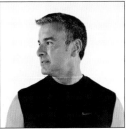

6. Seated Chest Stretch
Page 94

7. Scissors
Page 74

8. Seated Torso Twist
Page 80

9. Forearm Flip
Page 108

10. Neck Turn
Page 98

can slide into a shot without twisting your ankle.

Double up. Playing doubles is much easier on your knees and ankles because you only have to cover half the court. It also gives you a chance to finally perfect your net game.

The right racket. Modern materials have revolutionized racket design. Many pro shops will let you test new rackets before you buy and will help you find one that is easier on an arthritic wrist or hand or reverberates less on a stiff elbow. ■

10 Basketball

Perhaps with the success of a professional league of their own, women will learn what men have long known: Shooting baskets is great fun! And anyone can do it. You can just shoot around or you can ratchet it up to actually playing games. Shooting is tough on your neck, arms and shoulders. But the full game of basketball is tough on all of you. In fact, with its sprinting, jumping, pivoting and twisting, it is among the toughest sports if played full tilt. So if you are serious about maintaining a basketball habit with arthritis, you need a rigorous exercise routine like this one.

■ Strength Exercises

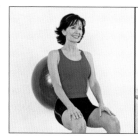

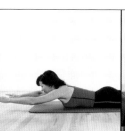

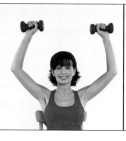

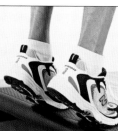

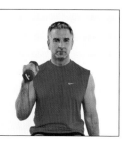

1. Ball Squat
Level 3, page 67

2. Superman
Level 2, page 91

3. Stair Heel Raise
Level 2, page 104

4. Overhead Dumbbell Press
Level 3, page 79

5. Hammer Curl
Level 2, page 111

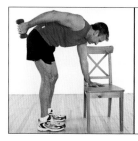

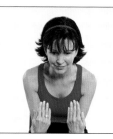

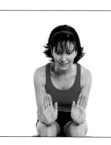

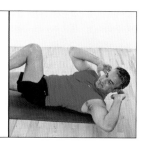

6. Triceps Kickback
Level 2, page 111

7. Wrist Curl
Level 1, page 116

8. Wrist Extension
Level 1, page 116

9. Advanced Bicycle
Level 3, page 85

everyday *secrets*

IN THE GAME

Again ... warm up! You'll be running, jumping, twisting. You'll be rebounding, shooting, dribbling. If you don't stretch your muscles in advance and get your blood flowing, you greatly increase your risk of injury or serious joint and muscle pain afterward.

Keep it mellow. The NBA may be getting more and more physical each year, but we advise you to leave full-contact play to the pros. Smart defenders know that by keeping their hands high and staying between the players they are guarding and the hoop, they make it awfully hard for their opponents to get off a shot. No roughhousing is necessary. Be strategic, not aggressive.

Monitor your energy. If you find yourself standing around during the action, head to the bench for a

Instructions

Again, we propose a three-part workout—aerobic, strengthening, then stretching—three times a week. For the aerobic component, do 20 to 30 minutes of brisk walking, cycling or light jogging, which mimics play on the court. Then do these 9 strengthening and 10 stretching moves. This part should take under 30 minutes. Start the strength exercises with one set of six repetitions. Try to hold your stretches for at least 15 seconds.

■ Flexibility Exercises

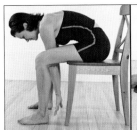 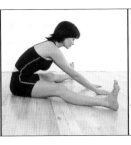 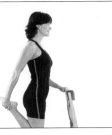 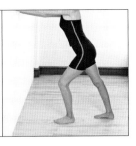

1. Seated Body Hang **Page 89**

2. Lying Total Body Stretch **Page 94**

3. Seated V **Page 57**

4. Standing Quad Stretch **Page 58**

5. Runner's Calf Stretch **Page 103**

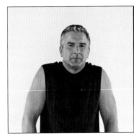 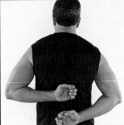 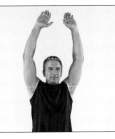 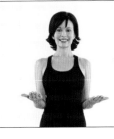 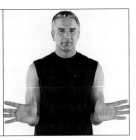

6. Shoulder Roll **Page 72**

7. Knuckle Rub **Page 73**

8. 'Good Morning' Exercise **Page 74**

9. Forearm Flip **Page 108**

10. Handshake Wrist Bend **Page 114**

rest. In a game, basketball players should be constantly on the go, getting clear for a pass or preparing to defend. Flat-footedness means you need a rest. Teams that win are the teams with energy, particularly in the fourth quarter.

Skip the game. There are many, many great basketball drills and games that are far easier on your joints than a formal game. Playing "21" from the foul line; having a game of Horse; even just lay-up drills or random shooting makes for a great time.

Make a clean shot. To improve your shooting, sometimes you just have to focus on setup and form, making sure your head and chest squarely face the basket, getting the ball into your favoured hand just before release and letting fly by flicking from the wrist, not pushing from the arms. ■

11 Swimming

No matter what your age or health, swimming is a delight. It feels good, it's fun and it's a wonderful way to exercise. Swimming mainly works your upper body. As a result, conditioning for swimming demands a lot of attention to range of motion and strength in the shoulders, back and chest, with a still-important nod to exercises for the hips, legs, ankles and feet.

■ Strength Exercises

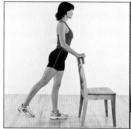 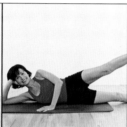 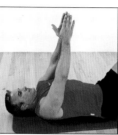 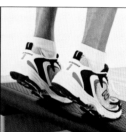 (first row)

1. Standing Hip Extension
Level 2, page 64

2. Side Thrust Kick
Level 3, page 67

3. Superman
Level 2, page 91

4. Chest Fly
Level 1, page 96

5. Stair Heel Raise
Level 2, page 104

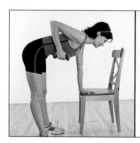 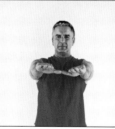 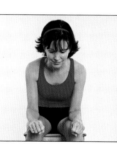 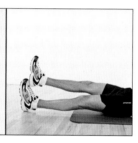

6. Bent Single Arm Row
Level 2, page 92

7. Around the World
Level 2, page 78

8. Wrist Rotation
Level 1, page 117

9. Flutter Kick
Level 2, page 83

---

everyday *secrets*

IN THE POOL

Position yourself. Getting through the water isn't merely a matter of generating power from your arms and legs. Instead, you'll slice surf easier (read: faster) by thinking of the shape your body makes as you move. Example: On a freestyle stroke, stretch your arm as far in front of you as possible after it enters the water (which the total body stretch will help you do) before pulling for power, to make your body longer and less resistant to the water.

Chafe at chopping. You're working hard, stirring up the water—but going nowhere. Don't mistake lots of effort for good exercise. You'll improve your efficiency and ultimately get a better cardiovascular workout if you focus on form, slicing your hand into the water on a freestyle stroke about

Instructions

Do these 9 strength exercises and 10 stretches two to three times per week to help prepare your body for swim time. As with the other routines, start the strength exercises with one set of six repetitions. Hold your stretches at least 15 seconds.

■ Flexibility Exercises

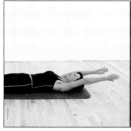 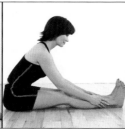 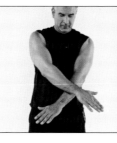 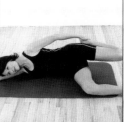

1. Lying Total Body Stretch
Page 94

2. Rocking Chair
Page 87

3. Straight-Leg Stretch
Page 57

4. Lying Quad and Hip Stretch
Page 58

5. Ankle Circle
Page 102

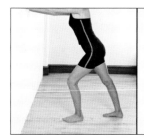 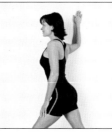 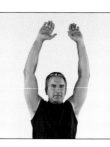 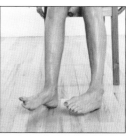 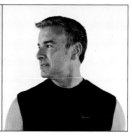

6. Runner's Calf Stretch
Page 103

7. Wall Stretch
Page 95

8. Scissors
Page 74

9. 'Good Morning' Exercise
Page 74

10. Neck Turn
Page 98

eight inches (20 cm) short of a complete arm extension and rotating your hips as you pull back.

Do a variety of strokes. To work muscles and joints from as many angles as possible, switch regularly from one stroke to another—freestyle, backstroke, breaststroke and sidestroke.

Be playful. A swimming pool is a wonderful thing—great for your muscles, your joints, your heart and your spirit. So don't make your pool time all hard work. Walking through the water, treading water, bouncing on the bottom, diving for pennies, playing catch with a ball, just floating contentedly on your back—all are wonderful for your body. Even standing still and talking with a friend is better for your health when done in a pool. ■

12 Skiing

Once you get the skiing bug, it never goes away. If weekend ski trips are the highlight of your winter, don't let arthritis slow you down. This program works the all-important hips, knees and back, while also exercising upper-body muscles and joints needed to propel or support yourself with a pole. A bonus: By getting your body in shape for skiing, you make falls and wipeouts less damaging.

■ Strength Exercises

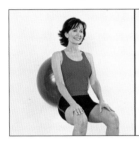

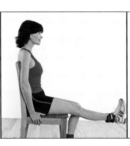

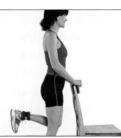

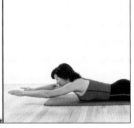

1. Ball Squat
Level 3, page 67

2. Around the World
Level 2, page 78

3. Seated Knee Extension
Level 2, page 66

4. Standing Knee Flexion
Level 2, page 64

5. Superman
Level 2, page 91

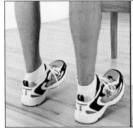

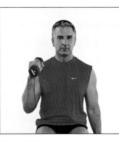

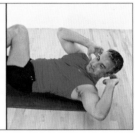

6. Heel/Toe Raise
Level 2, page 105

7. Triceps Kickback
Level 2, page 111

8. Hammer Curl
Level 2, page 111

9. Basic or Advanced Bicycle
Level 2 or 3 depending on variation, page 83 or 85

everyday secrets

ON THE SLOPES

Stay loose. If you take a spill on the slopes, you'll come out better if you keep your body relaxed rather than fighting the fall, which makes muscles tense and more prone to injury. Try to get your feet downhill as quickly as possible, especially on a steep slope, so you're better able to brake and absorb the force of further falling.

Take it easy. If downhill skiing becomes too much of a challenge, switch to cross-country skiing. It may not have the excitement of alpine skiing, but it is easier on the joints and a better aerobic workout.

Focus on lateral movement. Skiing demands lots of side-to-side movements that aren't natural in everyday life. So if you are serious about preventing soreness and

Instructions

When ski season approaches, we recommend you do this three-part exercise program to get ready. Three times a week is best, for at least a month prior to hitting the slopes. First, do a cardiovascular workout: 15 to 20 minutes of cycling or brisk walking (both level and on hills, if possible) or climb stairs to build leg endurance. Then do the following 9 strengthening and 7 stretching moves. This part should take under 20 minutes. Start the strength exercises with one set of six repetitions. Hold your stretches at least 15 seconds.

■ Flexibility Exercises

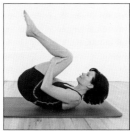 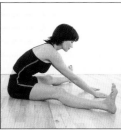 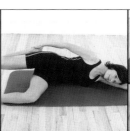 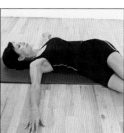 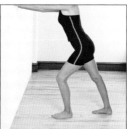

1. Rocking Chair	2. Seated V	3. Lying Quad and Hip Stretch	4. Pelvic Twist	5. Runner's Calf Stretch
Page 97	**Page 57**	**Page 58**	**Page 87**	**Page 103**

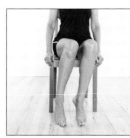 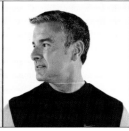

6. Seated Swivel	7. Neck Turn
Page 103	**Page 98**

avoiding injury, do sports or exercises that have you moving laterally. Even just a few minutes of shuffling sideways three or four times a week helps. Better is to line dance, play a little soccer with junior or get in some tennis a few times a week leading up to ski season.

Work on your balance. Ultimately, skiing is about your ability to keep your weight upright and centred as your lower body moves through a wide range of motion. Balance starts in the torso, so be sure to exercise your abs and lower back well prior to ski season. In addition, do anything you can to practice your sense of balance—from standing on one foot to balancing on your toes. ■

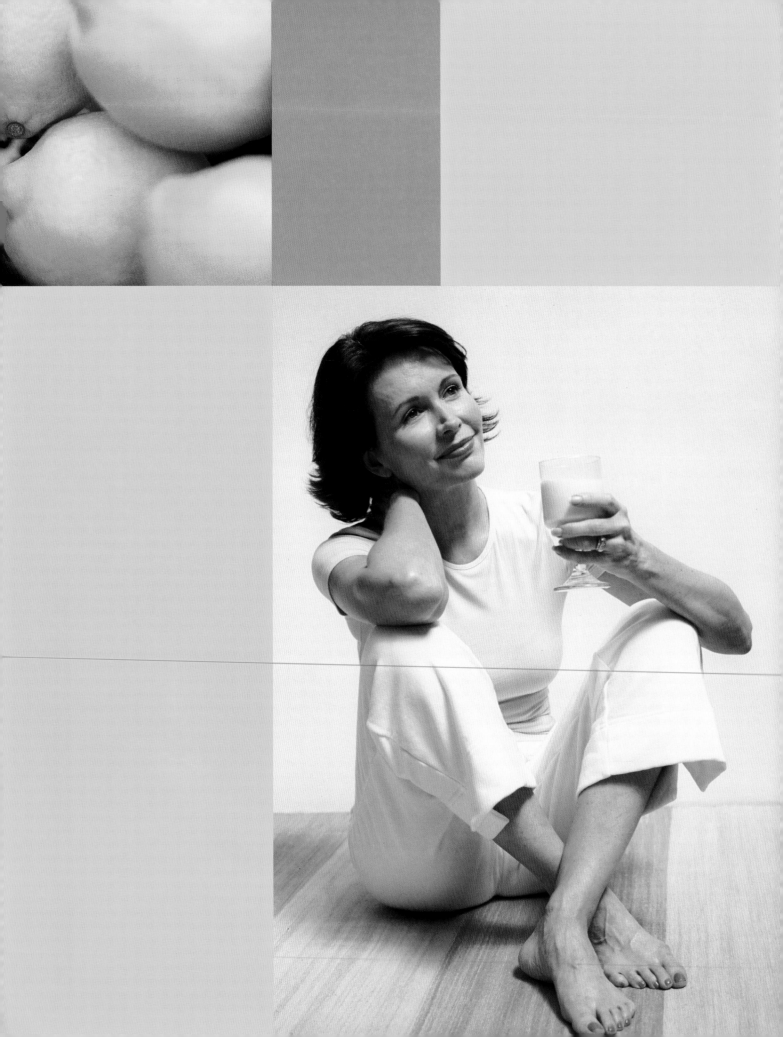

everyday food solutions

"You are what you eat" is one of the oldest phrases in the lexicon of moms. Yet the message is as important for people with arthritis as it is for candy-gobbling children. In the pages ahead, you will discover foods and supplements that can indeed help you achieve healthier, less painful joints. You'll also learn the universal secrets of eating to lose weight, which is one of the best ways to alleviate arthritis pain. And best of all, you will encounter a dazzling assortment of simple and delicious recipes, each one rich with the nutrients you need to overcome arthritis.

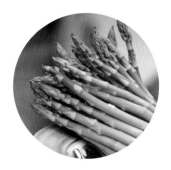

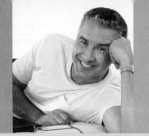
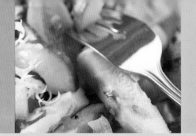

the best foods and supplements

Is there an arthritis diet? Your doctor would probably say no. Diet doesn't appear to affect arthritis to the same extent that it does heart disease, diabetes, some cancers and other illnesses and conditions. As a result, no one has worked up exact guidelines, backed by decades of studies, on eating to beat arthritis.

Does that mean diet doesn't matter? Far from it. Even though there's much more to learn, compelling evidence suggests that eating a healthy diet—and even specific types of food—may help relieve arthritis symptoms or prevent arthritis from becoming worse. Lack of consensus may make precise diet prescriptions difficult, but making reasonable dietary choices at the very least can complement your exercise goals and improve your overall health. Here's how good nutritional choices affect arthritis:

- Getting more of nutrients believed to play a role in controlling inflammation may help ease symptoms, especially for rheumatoid arthritis.

- Making up for nutritional deficiencies sometimes caused by arthritis may help prevent joints from deteriorating further.

- Nutritional supplements such as glucosamine show promise in shoring up arthritic joints, although you should be cautious about self-medicating your disease.

- Losing weight by making smart food choices (along with burning calories with exercise) takes some of the load off joints, easing pain and slowing degeneration, especially with osteoarthritis.

There are no guarantees and what works for you may not work for everyone with aching joints. But consider the possibilities: In one study from Denmark that controlled calories and boosted intake of arthritis-fighting foods, people who stuck out the diet showed significant improvements in morning pain and pain intensity overall, joint swelling and medication costs.

SIX Key Anti-Arthritis Nutrients

The basic goal of good nutrition is to get enough of everything—which is easy if you eat a balanced diet that includes lots of different foods. But these six nutrients appear to have special benefits for people with arthritis. None of these nutrients offer miracle cures and some appear to have more of an impact on arthritis than others. Bottom line: It's likely these nutrients help, getting more of them certainly won't hurt you and it's easy to work them into your daily eating without overhauling your diet. Recipes starting on page 217 will show you how.

1. Omega-3 Fatty Acids

They may sound technical and unappetizing, but it's worth savouring what omega-3s do for the body—especially the joints. Fatty acids are a family of special fats that the body needs but can't make for itself, so you have to get them from food. Once in the body, they collect in cells, where they help form hormone-like substances, called leukotrienes, that put the brakes on inflammation—a root cause of rheumatoid and, to a lesser extent, osteoarthritis. More than a dozen reliable studies suggest that increasing your intake of omega-3 fatty acids can help quell symptoms of rheumatoid arthritis, even if the fats don't slow progression of the disease.

The most important food source of omega-3s is cold-water fish like salmon, tuna, mackerel and trout. But you'll also find omega-3s in nuts and seeds, beans, soy foods, green leafy vegetables and cooking oils such as canola oil. Fish oil is not entirely benign: Taking large amounts in supplements can have side effects and eating too much fish raises health concerns. And cod liver oil? It is high in calories, has high amounts of vitamin A and may be heavy in cholesterol. Here's how to safely add omega-3s to your diet.

● **Switch from corn oil to canola oil.** Close relatives of the omega-3s are the omega-6s, fatty acids found in corn and other vegetable oils. While omega-3s (found in abundance in canola oil) are beneficial for your joints, omega-6s aren't: they make arthritis pain worse by promoting inflammation. They also compete with omega-3s in the body. So by switching your cooking oil, you boost your cells' usage of omega-3s and bring your body's fatty acids into better balance.

● **Consider omega-3 supplements.** To get omega-3s in the amounts used for many studies, you'd need to eat more fish than you can probably stomach—at least three servings every day. That makes taking fish oil supplements a viable alternative. But first, check with your doctor. On the whole, fish oil is safe, with mild side effects such as fishy burps. But omega-3 fatty acids also thin the blood, so you should be cautious if you're taking blood-thinning medications, including Aspirin.

● **Emphasize canned salmon and tuna.** It's not that they are richer in omega-3s than their fresh companions; it's that they are generally safer to eat. Health Canada has identified several types of predatory fish as rating above the official mercury guideline of 0.5 parts per million. These are mostly "gourmet fish," like fresh or frozen tuna, swordfish, shark and marlin. For these fish, Health Canada suggests keeping it to 150 g per week—or 150 g per month for women of childbearing age Canned tuna is exempt from this advisory; the cans tend to be packed with younger fish that haven't had as much time to accumulate toxins.

● **Say "no" if you have gout.** People with gout, a specific type of arthritis caused by excess uric acid, should avoid fish altogether because many types—including mackerel—contain purines, a building block for uric acid.

2. Vitamin C

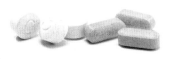

It's one of the most familiar of all nutrients, but vitamin C's role in joint health tends to be underappreciated. Vitamin C not only helps produce collagen, a major component of joints, but sweeps the body of destructive molecular byproducts known as free radicals, which are destructive to joints. Without vitamin C and other so-called antioxidant nutrients, free-radical damage to joints would be much worse. One of the best-known studies looking into vitamin C and arthritis, the Framingham osteoarthritis study, found that people whose diets routinely included high amounts of vitamin C had significantly less risk of their arthritis progressing. Points to bear in mind:

● **Drink OJ from frozen concentrate.** A prime source of vitamin C, orange juice is a favourite breakfast eye opener. While orange juice bought in the carton is healthy, OJ made from frozen concentrate is even better. According to recent research published by the American Dietetic Association, juice reconstituted from frozen concentrate has more vitamin C than fresh-squeezed juice after four weeks of storage. If you prefer no-fuss pourable products, buy juice three to four weeks before the expiration date and drink it within a week of opening.

● **Spread out intake.** Your body doesn't store vitamin C; rather, it takes what it needs from the bloodstream at any given time and flushes out the rest. So a megadose in the morning doesn't really do as much good as you would think. Rather, replenish your vitamin C stores throughout the day by sipping citrus drinks or eating C-rich fruits and vegetables such as strawberries or melon, broccoli or sweet peppers at meals.

● **Beware of megadoses.** Your body needs about 75 (for women) or 90 (for men) milligrams of vitamin C each day for basic bodily functions. For healing and antioxidant purposes, many people take much higher doses. Most people aren't affected by a few hundred milligrams of vitamin C, but once you get past 500 milligrams or so, you should check with your doctor. Some people develop digestive unrest when they megadose on the vitamin. In addition, high doses of vitamin C can raise blood levels of salicylate medications such as Aspirin and can also interfere with absorption of other nutrients.

3. Vitamin D

You can get vitamin D just from standing in the sun. That's because ultraviolet light converts pre-cursors of the vitamin in the body 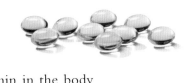 into a usable form. Many people with arthritis are D-deficient. Studies find that getting more vitamin D protects joints from osteoarthritis damage, probably because this nutrient is vital to the health of bones that support and underlie joints. Vitamin D also appears to play a role in production of collagen in joints themselves. Some suggestions:

● **Get into the sunlight.** You don't need to bake on the beach to get sun-stimulated vitamin D: The skin only needs 10 to 15 minutes of exposure two to three times a week to synthesize what it needs. Your usual outdoor walks, games, or yard work should fill your vitamin D needs.

● **Read your dairy labels.** Milk, from skim to homogenized, is a prime source of vitamin D because it is D-*fortified*. Check labels on other dairy products. Though domestic cheese, cream, ice cream, butter and yogourt often contain vitamin D, they're sometimes made with unfortified milk.

● **Beware of over-supplementing.** Vitamin D is a fat-soluble vitamin, which means excess amounts are stored in the body rather than immediately excreted. Large doses from high-potency supplements or multivitamins can build up and become toxic to soft tissues such as the kidneys and heart. Getting your D from foods and sunlight poses no such problems.

4. Vitamin E

Like vitamin C, this is an antioxidant vitamin that protects the body—including the joints—from the ravages of free radicals. Some of the same research showing that other nutrients protect against arthritis also indicates that vitamin E can help prevent joints from becoming worse, though E's effects appear more limited than those of vitamins C and D. Some suggestions for getting vitamin E into your body:

● **Try soybean oil.** In the omega-3 section, we suggested switching to canola oil, which is widely available and no more expensive than corn oil. To go one better, though, try finding and then cooking with soybean oil. Though vitamin E can be tough to get from eating prime sources such as wheat germ and avocados, it's easy to pick up in other foods when cooked in this E-rich oil. Bonus: Soybean oil is also a good source of omega-3 fatty acids.

● **Combine with fish oil.** Taking vitamin E together with fish oil seems to boost the body's ability to fight inflammation beyond what either nutrient would do on its own, according to two recent studies in animals at Loyola University in Illinois and the University of Buffalo. Be wary of heavy-duty supplements, however: Like fish oil, vitamin E thins the blood.

● **Compensate for cooking.** Whenever possible, eat E-rich foods raw—cabbage in coleslaw, for example. While a number of vegetables (including asparagus, Brussels sprouts and cabbage) contain small amounts of vitamin E, boiling can deplete food of as much as a third of its E content. Another option: Save cooking water, which retains leached nutrients and use it to moisten mashed potatoes or make soup or sauce.

Add nuts to your cereal, salads and snacks.
Sprinkling a quarter cup of almonds on your breakfast cereal or lunchtime salad will give you your daily requirement of vitamin E. Pumpkin and sunflower seeds, eaten as a snack or added to muffins, are another good source of vitamin E. Of course, dieters should be careful. Nuts are as high in calories as they are rich in nutrients, so weigh the benefits and drawbacks.

5. B Vitamins

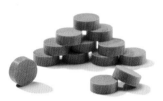

As cousin chemicals in the B-vitamin family of nutrients, vitamin B$_6$ and folate are also among the nutrients most likely to be lacking in people with arthritis. Part of this is due to deficiencies common population-wide—for example, one study found 90 percent of women don't get enough B$_6$ in their diet. But there's also evidence that the inflammation process eats up these B vitamins especially fast in people with rheumatoid arthritis—bad news for a variety of bodily functions, including the manufacturing of protein, the building block for tissues such as cartilage.

- **Double up.** When possible, eat foods that contain both vitamin B$_6$ and folate, such as spinach and fortified cereal. Otherwise, look to B vitamin sources for other arthritis-fighting nutrients. For example, in addition to being a rich source of B$_6$, tuna and sardines contain omega-3 fatty acids and fortified cottage cheese contains vitamin D. Bonus foods for folate include asparagus (vitamin E) and broccoli (vitamin C).

- **Take a multivitamin.** To ensure you get enough of these nutrients, consider taking a multivitamin that provides 100 percent of the recommended Dietary Allowance of 1 to 1.7 milligrams for B$_6$ and 0.4 milligrams for folate. (Look also for vitamin B$_{12}$, which works in tandem with folate.) But steer clear of high-dosage, single-nutrient supplements, which may pose risks of nerve damage.

6. Calcium

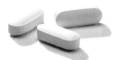

The issue with calcium, as with vitamin D, is bone health. Calcium has obvious importance to bones—more than 90 percent of the body's stores are contained in the skeleton and teeth. Getting too little calcium raises the risk of osteoporosis, a brittle-bone condition that accelerates if you have rheumatoid arthritis. All women (who are especially at risk) should get about 1,200 milligrams a day after age 50—about twice what's typical.

- **Drink milk; cook with milk.** You probably know that milk is a prime calcium source—but the same is true even for cooked foods made with

HOW TO TAKE YOUR VITAMINS

Taking a multivitamin is the obvious approach to getting enough nutrients, but you'll benefit from putting some thought into supplements. Here are a few points for getting the most from your daily dose:

■ **Take it with food**
The body is designed to absorb nutrients with real victuals and it's easier to remember a multivitamin when it's a regular part of your mealtime ritual.

■ **Keep your balance**
If you're taking a multi, don't take other specific vitamins unless your doctor recommends it.

■ **Keep up to date**
The vitamins lining store shelves don't seem perishable, but they do lose potency. Check expiration dates and don't buy more than you can use in the time allotted.

milk. So consider having pancakes or waffles (one large waffle may contain as much as 12 percent of your daily calcium requirement) at breakfast or lunch. For other meals, balance your diet with low-fat cheese as a topping for savoury fare such as chili or spaghetti.

● **Down it with D.** One reason vitamin D is so important to bone health is that it boosts the body's absorption of calcium—another reason to consume more D-fortified dairy, which contains both nutrients.

● **Go beyond the dairy case.** Milk and milk products aren't the only sources of calcium: It's also found in vegetables such as cauliflower, cabbage, Brussels sprouts, kale, kohlrabi, broccoli and turnip greens. These foods have less calcium than dairy products, but contain a form that's easier for the body to absorb. Other non-dairy calcium sources include omega-3-rich fish that have edible bones, such as salmon and sardines.

DO SOME FOODS MAKE ARTHRITIS WORSE?

Over the years, some arthritis sufferers have suspected that certain foods trigger symptoms or make them worse. Suspected triggers range from dairy, corn or cereals to the nightshade family of plants, which includes tomatoes, potatoes, peppers and eggplant. None of these ideas have been thoroughly studied, but

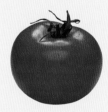

research suggests flare-ups people attribute to food are often actually due to some other cause.

So do your own test. If you suspect a food aggravates your arthritis, try eliminating the food for two to three weeks to see if you feel any better.

NINE Terrific Arthritis-Fighting Foods

It's easy to make arthritis-friendly nutrients part of a sensible daily diet because there's such a variety of them, covering virtually every food group. But with any nutrient, certain foods will always be richer sources than others. Below are super sources of the nutrients that battle arthritis best.

1. Salmon

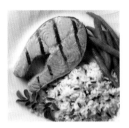

Salmon is among the richest sources of healthy fats, making it an ideal source of omega-3 fatty acids, especially because it's less likely than other cold-water fish to harbour high levels of toxic mercury. In addition to its fatty oils, salmon contains calcium, vitamin D and folate. Besides helping with arthritis, eating salmon may protect the cardiovascular system by preventing blood clots, repairing artery damage, raising levels of good cholesterol and lowering blood pressure.

● **Focus on freshness.** To avoid bacterial contamination, look for glossy fish that are wrapped to prevent contact with other fish. If you're buying fish whole, eyes should be clear and bright, not opaque or sunken and flesh should not be slimy or slippery. Cuts like steaks and fillets should be dense and moist. In all cases, flesh should be firm and spring back if you press it.

● **Use quickly.** Fresh fish spoils fast, so if you can't eat salmon within a day after purchase, double its shelf life by cooking it right away and storing it in the refrigerator. (It is delicious served cold with cucumbers and dill.)

● **Tame total fat.** While you want the beneficial omega-3s in fish oil, the fat in fish is also loaded with calories. To keep from adding still more calories during preparation, cook salmon using low-fat methods such as baking, poaching, broiling, or steaming and season with spices such as dill, parsley, cilantro, tarragon or thyme.

● **Cook by colour.** Following the rule of thumb for cooking fish—to wait until flesh is opaque white or light gray—is a tougher call with pink-hued salmon. To ensure doneness, cook salmon until it's opaque in its thickest part, with juices clear and watery and flesh flaking easily with the gentle turn of a fork.

2. Bananas

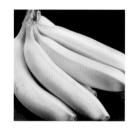

Bananas are perhaps best known for packing potassium, but they're also good sources of arthritis-fighting vitamin B_6, folate and vitamin C. What's more, this easily digested, dense fruit is a prime source of soluble fibre, an important part of your diet if you're trying to lose weight because it helps you feel full without adding calories.

● **Control ripeness.** Bananas are sweetest and easiest to digest when brightly yellowed to full ripeness. To hasten or prolong the period of perfection:
1. Put green bananas in a brown paper bag, which encourages natural gases from the bananas to speed the ripening process.
2. Put rapidly ripening fruits in the refrigerator, which turns the peel brown, but preserves the fruit inside.

● **Preserve pieces.** Bananas are wonderful additions to salads or desserts, but tend to turn brown faster than other ingredients. Try tossing bananas with a mixture of lemon juice and water—the acid will help preserve them.

● **Turn into drinks.** Bananas, particularly ripe ones, make great blender drinks. Combine a banana, a peach or some berries, a few millilitres of milk, a few millilitres of fruit juice and an ice cube and blend for a delicious, healthy drink that is jam-packed with arthritis-friendly nutrients.

3. Sweet Peppers

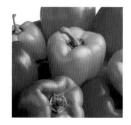

A single green pepper contains 176 percent of your daily needs for vitamin C—and colorful red and yellow varieties have more than double that amount. That makes them richer in C than citrus fruits, but sweet peppers are also excellent sources of vitamin B_6 and folate.

● **Lock in nutrients.** Store peppers in the refrigerator: The tough, waxy outer shell of bell peppers naturally protects nutrients from degrading due to exposure to oxygen, but you'll boost the holding power of chemicals in the skin by keeping them cold.

● **Separate seeds.** Whether cutting into crudités, tossing into salads, or stuffing whole, you'll want to remove tough and bitter-tasting seeds. They're easily cut when slicing, but when retaining an entire bell for stuffing, cut a circle around the stem at the top of the pepper, lift out the attached membranes and scoop remaining seeds and membranes with a thick-handled spoon.

● **Jam them in the juicer.** You might not think of peppers as juicer giants, but they can add zest to drinks made from other fruits and veggies.

● **Cook as a side dish.** Tired of the same old vegetables at dinner? Slice a pepper or two and do a fast sauté in olive oil, adding a pinch of salt, pepper and your favourite herb. The heat releases the sweetness, making sautéed peppers a wonderful counterpart to meats and starches.

4. Shrimp

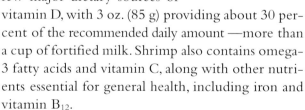

Taste and convenience make shrimp the most popular shellfish around. But shrimp also deserves acclaim as one of the few major dietary sources of vitamin D, with 3 oz. (85 g) providing about 30 percent of the recommended daily amount —more than a cup of fortified milk. Shrimp also contains omega-3 fatty acids and vitamin C, along with other nutrients essential for general health, including iron and vitamin B_{12}.

● **Select by senses.** When buying fresh raw shrimp, look for flesh that's moist, firm and translucent, without spots or patches of blackness. Then put your nose to work: Shrimp should smell fresh and not give off an ammonia-like smell, which is a sign of deterioration. If you're buying shrimp frozen, squeeze the package and listen: The crunch of ice crystals means the shrimp was probably partially thawed, then refrozen—a sign you should find another (less crunchy) package.

● **Eat or freeze.** When you get shrimp home, rinse under cold water and store in the refrigerator for up to two days. If you plan to store beyond that, stick to frozen shrimp, which will keep in the freezer for up to six months.

● **Cook quickly.** Overcooking makes shrimp tough, so it's best to cook it fast, boiling in water until shells turn pink and flesh becomes opaque, stirring occasionally. Rinse under cold water and serve alone, as part of a seafood chowder or chilled. Shrimp can also be broiled, grilled or stir-fried.

5. Soy Products

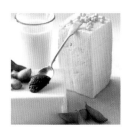

Once relegated to the shelves of health-food stores, soy products such as tofu and tempeh have reached the mainstream largely because they've been shown to have cardiovascular benefits. But soybeans also protect bones, thanks to compounds called isoflavones and significant amounts of both vitamin E and calcium. Long a staple of Asian diets, soy can also be found in soy milk—a boon for people who want to avoid lactose or cholesterol in regular milk.

● **Make the most of milk.** Use soy milk (now sold in many supermarkets next to cow's milk) for puddings, baked goods, cereal, shakes—just about anywhere you'd use regular milk. But don't mix it with coffee or other acidic foods, which tend to make soy milk curdle.

● **Try them whole.** Trust us: Whole soy beans, sprinkled with a little salt and pepper, are *delicious*. They look like large sweet peas but have an even gentler, milder flavour—nothing at all like the better known but more intimidating products like tofu. Check the freezer aisle for edamame (pronounced "ed-ah-MAH-may")—they come both in their pods or shelled. They cook up fast—about five minutes in boiling

water and two minutes in the microwave—and can be eaten hot or cold as snacks or appetizers or tossed into salads, stir-fries, casseroles or soups.

● **Give tofu a few more chances.** Many people don't know what to make of tofu. It's an odd colour for a vegetable-derived food (white), an odd texture (smooth and moist) and comes in an odd form (usually, a block). Get past all that. Tofu is easy to work with, extraordinarily healthy and takes on the flavours around it. Easy ideas: Drop half-inch (1-cm) cubes into most any soup; stir into tomato sauces, breaking it up into small pieces; or just cut into cubes, cover with chopped scallions and soy sauce and eat at room temperature as is.

6. Sweet Potatoes

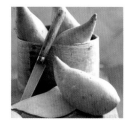

These tropical root vegetables (which are technically, not related to white baking potatoes) are such a nutritional powerhouse, they once topped a list of vegetables ranked according to nutritional value by the U.S.-based Center for Science in the Public Interest. Sweet potatoes are a rich source of vitamin C, folate, vitamin B_6 and dietary fibre, among other nutrients.

● **Buy fresh.** Though you'll benefit from eating sweet potatoes in any form, fresh potatoes are better than canned products, which are packed in a heavy syrup that leaches the vegetable's most valuable nutrients, including vitamins B and C.

● **Keep cool, not cold.** Store sweet potatoes someplace dark, dry and cool—preferably between 13 and 16°C (55 and 60°F)—but not in the refrigerator: Cold temperatures damage cells, causing the potato to harden and lose some of its nutritional value.

● **Maximize nutrients.** Eat cooked potatoes with their skin, which is an especially rich source of nutrients and fibre. Handle gently to avoid bruising, then bake or boil and serve with a touch of fat from butter, oil or another dish and some salt and pepper.

7. Cheese

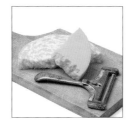

Hard or soft, fresh or ripened, cheese in all its variety is an excellent source of calcium for bones and protein for muscles and other joint-supporting tissues. Depending on type, cheeses (especially hard varieties such as cheddar and Colby) are also a good source of vitamin B_6 and folate. The sheer abundance of cheeses makes it easy to get more in your diet—by, for example, slicing hard cheeses onto crackers or grating them into casseroles or spreading soft cheeses such as cottage cheese or Brie onto fruits or vegetables.

● **Grease your grater.** When you have arthritis, grating cheese is hard enough without the grater becoming clogged. To make the job easier, give the grater a light coating of oil, which keeps the cheese from sticking and makes it easier to rinse the grater clean.

● **Lengthen shelf life.** Hard cheeses that are well wrapped and unsliced can last up to six weeks in the refrigerator. (Chilled soft cheeses are best used within a week.) To make cheese last even longer, throw it in the freezer, but expect thawed soft cheese to separate slightly and hard cheese to be crumbly—ideal for melting into casseroles and sauces but not as good for nibbling.

● **Let it warm.** Cheese tastes best when served at room temperature, so if you've been storing it in the refrigerator, take cheese out and let stand for an hour before serving to enjoy its full flavour.

● **Have a daily cheese platter.** Healthy eaters know that every dinner table should have a plate of fresh raw vegetables in addition to all the prepared foods. Consider adding a large hunk of cheese to the platter each night, along with a knife. Sitting there in front of you, it's hard to resist slicing a piece off a few times to round out the meal.

8. Lentils

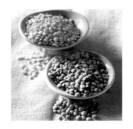

These dried legumes, with their rainbow of earthy hues, are prime sources of folate, with a single cup providing about 90 percent of your daily needs. But lentils also provide one of the richest plant-based sources of protein, contain large amounts of soluble dietary fibre and hold significant stores of vitamin B_6. These and other nutrients make lentils protect the body against heart disease and cancer in addition to arthritis.

● **Try a few soups.** Not many people know a lot of lentil recipes. The most common usage—soup—is probably the best place to start for those new to the food. You might be surprised at how easy and tasty lentil soups can be. Add cooked lentils to water or broth, chop in carrots, celery, onions and a lean meat, add some simple herbs and seasonings and you are well on your way to a great meal.

● **Buy in bags.** Though sometimes sold in bulk from bins, it's best to buy lentils in plastic bags, preferably with most beans shielded from light. Reason: Exposure to light and air degrades nutrients (especially vitamin B_6) and open bins invite contamination by insects.

● **Pick the best beans.** Even bagged products aren't pristine: Sort through lentils before you use them by spreading them on a baking sheet and picking out those that are shriveled or off-colour, along with any small stones that may have gotten mixed in. After that, there's no need to soak, but you should swish beans in a water-filled bowl, discard any floaters and rinse under cold water in a strainer before cooking.

● **Minimize gas.** Thoroughly drain lentils before eating or adding to other dishes: Beans are famous for causing gas due to sugars they contain that the body can't digest, but these sugars are soluble in water and leach out when lentils are cooked.

9. Green Tea

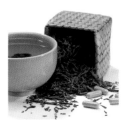

This mild, slightly astringent tea contains hundreds of powerful antioxidant chemicals called polyphenols and has been cited for helping prevent problems ranging from cancer to heart disease. But studies also suggest green tea may help prevent or ease symptoms of rheumatoid arthritis. In one study of induced arthritis in mice, green tea cut the disease onset rate almost in half and follow-up studies by the same researchers, at Ohio's Case Western Reserve University, show promise in humans.

- **Boil water briskly.** Tea tastes best when water is at the boiling point, which allows tea to release its flavourful compounds quickly. Water that's cooler than that tends to release flavours more slowly, weakening the tea.
- **Keep steeping short.** Let tea steep in hot water for about three minutes—and no longer than five. This brief steeping time allows tea to acquire a full-bodied flavour and release its nutrients, but withholds compounds that make tea taste bitter.
- **Get a bag bonus.** Tea purists favour the fresher flavour of loose tea, but some experts suggest that tea bags release more beneficial nutrients because smaller, ground-up particles expose more of the tea leaves' surface area to hot water.

TAKE THE TEA—DUMP THE DECAF

One study presented to a recent meeting of the American College of Rheumatology confirmed tea's arthritis-taming benefits: Older women who consumed three or more cups a day had a **60 percent lower risk of developing rheumatoid arthritis** than other women.

But just as remarkable was a tandem finding that women who drank four or more cups of decaffeinated coffee a day appeared to double their risk of developing RA.

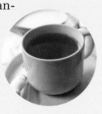

TWELVE Supplements to Be Aware Of

Anyone suffering from a chronic, painful condition such as arthritis is a prime target for sham treatments and there's no shortage of over-the-counter remedies and herbs that claim they'll make your life "normal" again. But while it's smart to be skeptical, studies find that some remedies show promise for relieving pain and restoring mobility. Few supplements have been studied rigorously either for effectiveness or safety, however, so it's best to explore supplements under the watchful eye of your medical support team.

Keep in mind that quality and purity of supplements can vary tremendously and always check with your doctor about side effects and drug interactions before starting to take any supplement regularly.

What follows here are details of 12 arthritis products you could see at stores, discover through advertisements on the Internet, or hear about through word of mouth. Unlike the nutrients we've just covered, we are not advocating you take any of these. Rather, study the information, consult with your doctor, and be aware that not every supplement is safe, appropriate, or effective for you.

1. Chondroitin Sulfate

Chondroitin sulfate—usually in combination with glucosamine—has been a popular arthritis remedy for years. But promising studies suggest that each of these supplements by itself may be effective at easing pain and improving joint function. Chondroitin is a natural component of human cartilage, but supplements are derived from cows or pigs. It's thought to ease symptoms of osteoarthritis by drawing fluid into joints to make them more supple and by preventing enzymes from breaking down cartilage. More than a dozen studies, taken together, suggest it has benefits. A U.S. study of Chondroitin Sulfate and Glucosamine funded by the National Institutes of Health found that the benefits to those suffering from only moderate OA pain were negligible, though those suffering from severe pain reported encouraging results.

Chondroitin appears safe, but it may affect blood sugar and thin the blood, so approach it cautiously if you have diabetes or take anticoagulant medications. Don't expect instant results: Even people who say it works find that chondroitin can take as long as two to four months to have an effect. Typical dosing for chondroitin is 1,200 mg a day divided into two or three equal amounts.

2. Collagen

Of two types of supplements that fall under this category, the most promising is collagen II, a natural component of cartilage. Usually made from animals such as chickens or cows, low-dose collagen II supplements are thought to relieve pain and stiffness from inflammation due to rheumatoid arthritis. One theory holds that introducing small amounts of supplemental collagen into the body causes attacking immune system cells to develop tolerance for your own collagen, making the immune system less likely to inflict more damage. Enough studies have suggested a positive effect from low doses that the National Institute of Arthritis and Musculoskeletal and Skin Diseases (NIAMS) in 1999 launched a collagen II trial, which is currently in phase II. Pending the trial's results, collagen II generally appears safe unless you have an allergy to chicken or eggs. Dosage recommendations vary widely, but best results in studies so far have been from extremely small amounts: The NIAMS study is using between 30 and 130 mcg a day. But supplements may not be necessary: You can also get collagen II from chicken soup.

Another type of collagen is collagen hydrolysate, sometimes known as gelatin, which is made by boiling the bones and skin of animals such as cows and pigs. Products containing gelatin have been promoted for arthritis based on the idea that amino acids in gelatin help repair and maintain joints. In one preliminary study, a powdered supplement containing gelatin, vitamin C and calcium improved pain, stiffness and mobility, but on the whole, claims for gelatin's benefits aren't well supported in the scientific literature. Still, though collagen hydrolysate may cause gastrointestinal trouble, it generally appears safe in typical doses of 10 grams.

3. CMO

This fatty substance, formally known as cetyl myristoleate, has been shown in an American study to prevent arthritis in mice (from which it's derived). Supplement makers have seized on this finding to bolster claims that CMO regulates the immune response responsible for conditions such as RA, fibromyalgia and ankylosing spondylitis. But how it may work is largely a mystery, and there's no good evidence that it is effective in humans. The American Arthritis Foundation notes that research establishing safe dosage is lacking and warns that some CMO promoters suggest you stop using doctor-prescribed arthritis medications to avoid blocking the effects of the supplement—a dangerous practice. For these reasons, many doctors recommend staying away from CMO and Health Canada has not approved it for sale.

4. Devil's Claw

The root of this herbaceous plant (named for the hooklike bumps on its fruit), is a traditional African pain reliever and a popular arthritis remedy. Its active ingredient, harpagoside, is thought to be an anti-inflammatory agent—the basis for thinking devil's claw may help relieve pain and ease symptoms of arthritis, particularly RA. Much of the research on devil's claw has been done in Europe, where Germany's Bundesinstituts für Arzneimittel und Medizinprodukte (Federal Institute for Drugs and Medical Devices) reports most studies to be poorly conducted and findings to be mixed. One of the best studies, however, found devil's claw to be effective against arthritis pain, though it's unclear whether the herb actually reduces inflammation or works in some other way.

Devil's claw, which comes in capsules, teas and tinctures, appears to be safe even in doses above the 2 and 4 grams typically recommended. It's best taken between meals because stomach acids that peak after eating may hinder its effects. Caveats: Be careful if you have ulcers or diabetes, take blood thinners or are pregnant: Devil's claw can stimulate the gastrointestinal tract and uterine wall and may interfere with certain medications.

5. DHEA

Not a nutrient or herb, DHEA (dehydroepiandrosterone) is the body's most abundant androgen—a type of steroid hormone that's used to make other hormones, including testosterone and estrogen. People with rheumatoid arthritis have been found to have low levels of DHEA, prompting speculation that taking more in supplements might ease RA symptoms, especially since androgens are known to inhibit the body's immune response. Does DHEA work? So far, there's no direct evidence it actually controls rheumatoid arthritis, but a number of studies suggest it relieves joint pain and inflammation in women with lupus, another joint disease caused by immune system attack.

Purity and dosage (which are frequently iffy with supplements) are particularly important with DHEA because it has potentially serious side effects. These may include raising risks of endometrial cancer and prostate cancer and lowering amounts of "good" HDL cholesterol in blood. More immediate hormone-related side effects may include hair growth on the face and body, acne, deepening of the voice and menstrual irregularities. In Canada, DHEA is considered a drug, specifically an anabolic steroid. It is a controlled substance and is only available by prescription.

6. GLA

Gamma-Linolenic acid—an active ingredient in evening primrose oil, black currant oil and borage oil—is a fatty acid that helps the body produce anti-inflammatory prostaglandins. Though it hasn't been thoroughly researched, several good, small studies find GLA can help ease joint pain or stiffness from rheumatoid arthritis by as much as a third. In one study, almost three-quarters of people with RA who took evening primrose oil were able to cut back on their NSAID medications. The U.S. Arthritis Foundation says that such findings make GLA worth a try.

GLA's long use as a remedy for RA (and other problems such as eczema and diabetic neuropathy) provides a long safety record in which there appear to be no serious side effects. The main drawback may be that,

depending on the type of oil you take and the amount of GLA per capsule or tablet, you could need dozens of pills to reach recommended doses between 1.8 and 2.8 grams a day. Look for high-dose products, but check with your doctor before starting a regimen: Oils containing GLA can thin the blood.

7. Glucosamine

Like chondroitin, glucosamine is a natural component of your own joints, but supplements get it from animals—in this case, shellfish. Glucosamine also appears to be one of the most effective natural remedies for shoring up degenerating joints. One of the most recent well-controlled studies of glucosamine found that taking supplements for three years held back progression of osteoarthritis and relieved symptoms by as much as 25 percent. Numerous studies over the past two decades have found that glucosamine relieves arthritis pain just as well as NSAIDs like ibuprofen—sometimes better—with fewer side effects. It's not entirely clear how glucosamine works, but it's thought to provide joints with extra proteins that actually build or maintain tissue. It may also act as anti-inflammatory agent.

As with chondroitin, glucosamine can take as long as two months to produce results, but appears to be safe in typically recommended doses of 1,500 mg, which you can find in capsules, tablets, liquid and powder that you mix into a drink. Though it's worth being wary of glucosamine if you're allergic to shellfish, it generally appears safe, with few side effects beyond mild gastrointestinal problems (which you may be able to remedy by switching to another brand). Check with your doctor, however, if you have high cholesterol, triglycerides or blood sugar—glucosamine may raise levels of all three.

8. MSM/DMSO

MSM (methylsulfonylmethane) is a relatively recent arrival on the supplement scene, but DMSO (dimethyl sulfoxide), from which it's derived, has been touted as an arthritis remedy for decades. DMSO is an extremely versatile solvent that's used both for industrial purposes (it's in paint thinner and antifreeze) and medical applications (it's used to protect organs during transplantation, among other things). Though it is routinely used as an arthritis treatment in some countries, it is not approved for arthritis care in Canada. The results from a mid-90s trial in Germany that showed benefits from rubbing a topical DMSO gel onto painful areas have yet to be reproduced in North America.

Enter MSM, which has been touted as the active ingredient in DMSO—only safer. Proponents say it's an anti-inflammatory that can ease symptoms of rheumatoid arthritis and some studies have suggested a benefit in mice. But there's no scientific evidence that it works in people or that it's safe.

9. SAM-e

Popularly known as "Sammy," S-adenosylmethionine is a naturally occurring chemical with dozens of functions in the body. Often used as an antidepressant, it's also reputed to rebuild cartilage, hinder inflammation and ease pain in people with osteoarthritis. It's long been available in Europe, where multiple studies have suggested SAM-e improves joint symptoms. In one large study, about 80 percent of arthritis sufferers taking SAM-e reported less pain. Other studies find it has pain-relieving effects comparable to many NSAIDs, though SAM-e works more slowly.

SAM-e generally appears safe in both human and animal studies. A typical full dose is 400 mg three times a day, which may be reduced to 200 mg when symptoms begin to improve. (Avoid high doses, which can cause gastrointestinal problems.) Though SAM-e isn't found in food, you may be able to boost your own natural production by eating green, leafy vegetables and other foods high in folate, which helps the body make SAM-e. Be sure to tell your doctor if you start taking supplements, especially if you're on antidepressants, which may interact with SAM-e.

10. Shark Cartilage

If osteoarthritis makes you lose cartilage, why not replace it by eating more? That's one way to explain why taking supplements of cartilage ground from sharks or other animals might fight arthritis. But shark cartilage

Other Armouries of ARTHRITIS-FIGHTING NUTRIENTS

Omega-3 fatty acids
pecans
black beans
flaxseed

Vitamin C
broccoli
strawberries
tomatoes

Vitamin D
eggs
mushrooms
tuna

Vitamin E
spinach
asparagus
lobster

Vitamin B6
chicken
avocado
cantaloupe
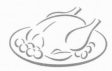

Folate
corn
peas
kidney beans
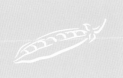

Calcium
sardines
turnip greens
black-eyed peas
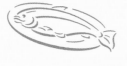

also contains collagen II, chondroitin sulfate and calcium—all of which play a role in maintaining healthy joints or show promise in relieving arthritis symptoms. Preliminary animal and lab studies suggest that shark cartilage may indeed have anti-inflammatory and analgesic effects, but no well-controlled studies in people have yet shown it to have any impact on arthritis. Likewise, little is known about how much shark cartilage in capsules, tablets or powder you should take, though per-pill doses on the market range from 250 mg to 750 mg. The most common side effects include gastrointestinal problems such as nausea and vomiting, but shark cartilage has also been known to cause low blood pressure, dizziness, high blood sugar and fatigue.

11. Stinging Nettle

Approved by the German medical establishment for treating prostate problems in men, supplements made from the stalklike stinging nettle plant are also said to reduce inflammation and ease pain from arthritis. In folk medicine, the irritating leaves of the plant were rubbed on the site of pain, which probably either triggered an anti-inflammatory reaction at the site or simply overrode one form of discomfort with another. Today fresh leaves have been replaced by extracts in capsules, teas and tinctures designed to ease pain without irritation. Research suggests nettle supplements may work. One German study found that peo-ple who took a quarter dose of a prescription NSAID along with stinging nettle reduced pain from arthritis just as much as people who took the full drug dose. Other studies also find that taking stinging nettle can reduce your need for pain medication.

To use stinging nettle, take 1 to 4 mL of tincture or make tea three times a day. To make tea, mix two teaspoonfuls of finely cut herb in water, boil, steep for 10 minutes, strain and drink one cup.

12. Thunder God Vine

For thousands of years, extracts from roots of this Asian plant (also called *lui kong teng*) have been used in traditional Chinese medicine to reduce pain and inflammation that go hand-in-hand with autoimmune diseases such as RA. Now science is catching up: A 2002 study funded by the National Institute of Arthritis and Musculoskeletal and Skin Diseases found that 80 percent of people with rheumatoid arthritis who took thunder god vine extract showed rapid improvement in their symptoms with minimal side effects. Lab and animal studies suggest the vine hinders production of chemicals that contribute to inflammation.

Though studies into the use and effectiveness of thunder god vine use extracts of 30 mg, Western science has not yet established guidelines for safe doses, meaning that this supplement is something on the horizon, rather than a viable option at the moment.

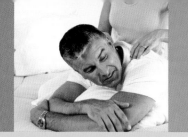
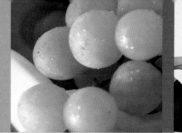
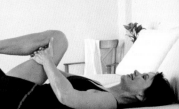

weight loss and arthritis

Losing weight: It's a North American obsession. Bookstores, magazine racks, television talk shows, infomercials, billboards—you can't escape the latest diets, the outlandish promises, the ubiquitous before-and-after photos. Or get through a day without encountering a weight-loss conversation. Many people are disgusted by it all. Why can't we just accept ourselves as we are?

The disgust may be justified. The marketing of weight loss has gotten out of control to the point that a Canadian, U.S. and Mexican trilateral charter on weight loss fraud has started to crack down on it all, and cities like Madrid have banned the use of underweight models in fashion shows. But just because the marketing is excessive doesn't mean the goal of weight loss isn't desirable. It is, in just so many ways.

Weight loss isn't merely about vanity; it's about health. Particularly for people with arthritis, achieving a healthy weight can make all the difference in reducing pain and halting the advance of the disease. The primary reason is obvious: Carry around less weight and you put far less stress and strain on your joints.

Being overweight with arthritis can become a vicious circle. Loading joints—especially knees—with extra pounds causes more pain and decreases mobility. That typically makes you cut back on physical activity, which in turn contributes to even more weight gain.

If you've started getting more physical activity to build strength and endurance, you've already taken a giant step toward breaking the cycle of increasing weight, pain and disability. But most overweight people (and their doctors) recognize that exercise alone won't pare pounds. Instead, you need to combine your calorie-burning activity with diet control.

Losing weight can seem daunting, particularly with all the conflicting approaches and products being pushed at us. But the most effective diet tactics are deceptively simple. Better yet, they work best when you apply them over time rather than making a drastic overhaul of your current eating habits.

There's no doubt the changes are worth the effort. One of the most recent studies connecting weight and arthritis, a 2003 study of twins in Britain, found that about 56 percent of osteoarthritis is due to being overweight—a more significant role than genetics. But the fatness factor works in reverse as well, according to the Framingham osteoarthritis study, which found that dropping just two units on the body mass index scale (about 11 lbs or 5 kilos for most people) cuts your risk of pain and stiffness by half.

Overweight and OA

Piling on extra pounds is now recognized as a major cause of osteoarthritis. And judging by recent surveys showing that more than half of all North Americans are overweight, it may be the most important cause of all. In particular, obesity can cause OA of the weight-bearing joints—the knees and, to a lesser extent, the hips. But it is also associated with a greater risk of OA in other joints as well, including the back, ankles, big toes and hands.

The pressure of pounds.
When you think about it, obesity's role in causing OA—or in aggravating symptoms in

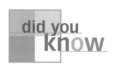

Eliminating obesity in Canada would lower the incidence of OA of the knee by 25 to 50 percent, and reduce the incidence of OA of the hip by 25 percent or more.

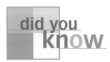
people who already have the disease—makes all too much sense. The protective cartilage that covers the ends of the bones in a joint is just a few millimetres thick. Years of carrying around spare kilos puts extra pressure on the knees and other weight-bearing joints, grinding down cartilage to the point that bone rubs against bone and giving rise to the pain and stiffness of OA. In people who already have OA, being overweight can speed up cartilage loss and cause the disease to worsen.

Studies have documented the overweight-arthritis link. They've followed groups of people over several years, keeping close tabs on their weight and whether they developed OA. One study involved more than 1,000 women age 45 to 64 who lived in London; 58 out of the 67 women with OA in one knee returned for a follow-up X-ray two years later. Of the 32 clearly overweight women,

15—or nearly half—had by then developed OA in their other knee as well; but only one of the 10 normal-weight women had gone on to develop OA in her other knee.

Cutting Through the Controversies

Which diets take weight off best is the subject of heated scientific debate. No wonder: According to Statistics Canada, 59.2 percent of Canadians are overweight or obese—a figure that has climbed steeply in the last decade and continues to rise. But it's important to recognize that, though there's much haggling over details (albeit important ones), there's also general agreement on a number of critical points.

For starters, weight-loss advice for decades has focused on cutting fatty foods, mainly because doing so is an important way to cut risks of cardiovascular disease. As a result, "the public has come to think that eating too much fat is the only cause of overweight and obesity, which isn't true," says Robert Murray, M.D., who is associated with the Borden Center for Nutrition and Wellness at Ohio State University and is a medical director at Ross Laboratories, a division of Abbott Laboratories. In fact, guidelines from

WHAT'S YOUR CALORIE BUDGET?

Everybody's calorie needs are different, based on factors such as weight and activity levels. Your doctor or dietitian can help you figure exactly how many calories you should be eating every day, but there's also a way to come up with your own ballpark estimate. Here's how:

1.
Multiply your weight by 10. This provides a rough idea of how many calories your body needs when resting.

2.
Get an idea how many calories you typically burn with activity by using the following scale. If you're completely sedentary, give yourself 300. If you're moderately active, give yourself 500. And if you're very active, give yourself 700.

3.
Add the numbers from steps 1 and 2. This is approximately how many calories you need and can take in every day without putting on extra pounds.

the U.S. National Heart, Lung and Blood Institute (NHLBI) state that reducing dietary fat alone "is not sufficient for weight loss." Instead, the consensus from NHLBI says the real issue is reducing calories. A key to doing it: Cutting back not just on fat but also on carbohydrates, which many people mistakenly believe are virtually harmless when it comes to weight loss.

Today the pendulum has swung all the way to the other side: Nearly every new weight-loss program focuses on a low-carbohydrate eating. The science of high-protein, low-carb diets is complicated, having to do with the way your body processes nutrients, the nature of your metabolism and the energy stores from which your cells draw their fuel.

But at the end of the day, no matter which diet you use, the basic problem is energy balance. To lose weight, you need to take in less energy (that is, calories) than you burn—by eating less, exercising more... or both. Even a small tip of the calorie balance can make a big difference over time. According to the NHLBI, the ideal diet leaves you with an average energy deficit of at least 500 calories a day (less than the amount in two peanut butter cookies), with a goal of dropping just a bit each week (500 grams or 1 pound). When weight loss plateaus, as it usually does after three or four months, exercise becomes especially important for maintaining losses and building muscle, which burns calories more efficiently than flab. Your weight loss may come slowly with these methods, "but if you're consistent, you'll make progress," says Murray.

How many of your calories should be fat versus carbohydrate? "What works best for you ultimately depends on what you can stick with and still reduce calories," says Murray. "Calories are where you make your stand." He recommends cutting back first on foods with heavy calories but little nutrition, such as cookies and ice cream—though you can indulge in them for the occasional treat or celebration. Next, get more vegetables (staples of both low-fat and low-carb diets) and whole-grain foods: They're rich in nutrients and fibre, which fills you up and keeps cravings at bay. Beyond that, Murray says, "there are a lot of ways to use food strategically."

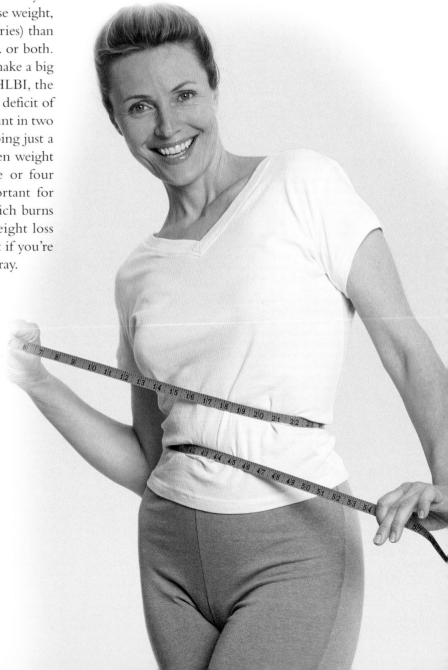

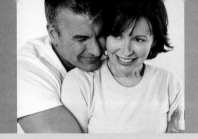
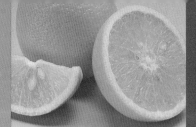
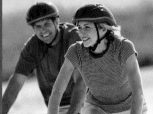

the upside of slimming down

The good news is that overweight people who lose weight can prevent OA of the knee from occurring. This was first demonstrated in a study published in 1992—the first ever to show that OA was potentially preventable. And the weight loss didn't need to be dramatic: By losing just 5 kilograms (11 pounds) over a 10-year period, the study found, an overweight woman could reduce her risk for developing OA of the knee by 50 percent.

The vicious cycle. When it comes to OA, being overweight is notorious for pushing patients down that long and slippery slope paved with increasingly more severe symptoms. Once people develop arthritis, there are often reasons—many of them totally understandable—why patients continue to put on weight or can't take it off. Arthritis sufferers frequently become depressed, which can lead to overeating and even more weight gain. In addition, someone with stiff, sore joints tends to prefer the couch to the track, leading to more weight gain and even worse pain and disability.

And it goes beyond arthritis. Being overweight can increase your risk for developing many other health problems as well—high blood pressure, adult-onset diabetes, heart disease, and several types of cancer, including prostate and colorectal cancer.

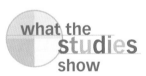

what the studies show

Studies have shown that fibre-rich foods are a natural appetite suppressant. Because they take up more room in your stomach than other foods, you feel fuller faster. Fiber is slower to digest, so it keeps hunger at bay longer. And most fiber-rich foods simply take more time to chew (think granola vs. doughnut), so your brain has more time to register that you've had enough—before you've had too much.

Canada's Food Guide: Eat to Lose

Healthy eating involves much more than just playing bean counter and adding up long lists of calories you consume. The idea is not only to lose weight if you need to but also to eat the right kinds of foods: those that are low in fat and high in beneficial nutrients such as fibre and vitamins.

Optimally, this approach to eating will be not only effective but also practical—an eating strategy that you can stick with over the long haul without feeling deprived or bored.

One eating approach does meet those requirements, but it doesn't receive the hype of the Zone Diet, the Atkins Diet, or the other highly touted fad diets that publishers trot out with regularity. It's known as Canada's Food Guide.

Losing it for good. The Food Guide is intended to guide you in choosing the types of foods to eat each day. It has two crucial advantages over its flashier (and flash-in-the-pan) competitors: You'll have a better chance of sticking with it for life, and nutrition experts regard it as the healthiest eating strategy yet devised.

Sticking with the Food Guide can help people with OA lose weight if necessary and then maintain the healthy weight they've achieved. Equally important, it can help you ward off or reduce your risk for developing cancer, heart disease, diabetes, hypertension, and other health problems associated with being overweight. The diet accomplishes these aims by emphasizing the three factors that are key to healthy eating: balance, variety, and moderation.

A Guide—Not a Diet

Over 50 million North Americans are dieting at any one time—and you may well be among them. If so, your hopes of slimming down will almost inevitably end in disappointment.

Extensive research and surveys of dieters themselves all show that any reducing diet or commercial diet program can produce significant weight loss—and even produce it rapidly. But the ultimate goal is to keep that weight off, and the vast majority of dieters are not able to do that. Almost inevitably, they promptly regain all the weight they lose on diets.

Focus on food. The Food Guide is not a diet but a healthful approach to eating. It doesn't focus on calories but emphasizes the food groups that are best for long-term good health: grains, fruits, and vegetables. These foods are high in health-promoting vitamins, minerals, and other nutrients and low in saturated fat, cholesterol, and calories.

⇒ BONING UP: It's best to get your nutrients from whole food rather than supplements. Foods contain a host of other beneficial substances that can be critical to minimizing your symptoms.

Not surprisingly, pursuing the Guide's recommendations will likely mean reducing your calorie intake and losing weight in the process—and running an excellent chance of maintaining that weight loss.

Using the Guide

If you include the number of servings of food recommended in Canada's Food Guide, you'll have little appetite left for the chips and junk food. Still, the Guide does provide you with enough latitude to keep your diet interesting. The key is to make the right choices within each food group. Your daily nutrient intake should lean heavily on fruits and veggies (between seven and 10 servings per day for adults), with grains coming up a very close second (six to eight servings). Dairy meats, or alternatives should clock in at two or three servings per day.

Healthy choices. For fruit, a good approach it to put it where you can see it. People are more likely to eat

ANTIOXIDANTS FOR ARTHRITIS

Findings from the landmark Framingham study indicate that the antioxidant vitamins C, E and beta carotene help to prevent the progression of osteoarthritis. Antioxidants help to neutralize free radicals, chemicals continually formed within cells during normal metabolism that can damage cartilage and possibly cause inflammation as well.

So what are the best sources of antioxidants? Fruits and vegetables, of course. Here is a cheat sheet on how to maximize your daily antioxidant intake. Eat...

- Red grapes rather than green or white varieties
- Red and yellow onions instead of white
- Cabbage, cauliflower, and broccoli raw or lightly cooked
- Garlic raw and crushed
- Fresh and frozen vegetables rather than canned ones
- Microwaved vegetables instead of boiled and steamed ones
- The deepest, darkest green leafy vegetables
- Pink grapefruit instead of white grapefruit
- Whole fruits rather than juices
- Fresh and frozen juices instead of canned ones
- The deepest orange carrots, sweet potatoes, and pumpkins

fruit that's in a bowl on a counter than in a refrigerator. As for grains, eat mostly whole grains that are high in fibre. Because most fibre leaves the body undigested, your body doesn't absorb the calories it contains. Dairy? Lower-fat varieties provide the same beneficial nutrients as their full-fat brethren, without the fat and calories. As for meats, trim the fat and choose leaner, choice cuts rather than prime. For chicken and its ilk, white meat is lower in fat than dark, and removing the skin is a foolproof way to decrease the fat.

Sweet somethings. Canada's Food Guide includes a section on Oils and Fats, which states that it's best to stick with oils like canola, olive or soy, and to limit your use of butter, hard margarine, lard and shortening.

Calories are calories, right? Wrong: researchers now know that not all calories are the same: Calories from fat are the worst, since they are more efficiently stored as fat in the body than are calories from carbohydrates or protein. And a diet high in fat—especially the saturated fat found in animal products—raises blood cholesterol levels and increases the likelihood of developing certain cancers.

⇒ BONING UP: Regular exercise can be extremely effective in weight control. In fact, study after study shows that dieting alone can help people lose weight—but that exercise is needed to keep it off.

What to do? Well, by making some minor substitutions, you can significantly reduce the amount of fat in your diet. The table below illustrates the differences in fat among foods that are otherwise similar. To single out one example: Pretzels and potato chips are both salty snacks, but 30 g (1 oz) of chips contains 11 times more total fat than an equal weight of pretzel twists.

Make Changes Slowly

Changing something as basic as what you eat—tofu instead of steak, say—can be difficult indeed. You're most likely to succeed over the long term if you proceed gradually. A few tips:

- If you use cream in your coffee, switch to homogenized milk for a few weeks, then to 2% milk, then to 1% and finally to skim milk.

- Eat more slowly. You'll find that you feel satisfied with smaller portions.
- Move meat, chicken, and fish from the centre of your plate and make vegetables the largest serving.
- Cut recipe amounts of meat in half; use only lean meats (look for round or loin on the package), and fill in the lost bulk with shredded vegetables, legumes, pasta, grains, or other low-fat items.
- When you go to the supermarket, buy a fruit or vegetable that you've never tried before.
- When you leave for work or for a day's outing, bring your food along with you to avoid buying fat-filled fast food.

Watch Those Portions!

Nutrition experts all seem to agree: North Americans have an exaggerated idea of what size a serving should be. Restaurants especially deserve blame for implanting the idea of supersizing in the minds of consumers. So, the trend has been toward consuming larger food portions, especially of foods rich in fat and sugar. At the same time, the collective waistline has been expanding, suggesting an increasing need to control portion sizes if we are to win the battle of the bulge.

This distorted notion of serving size not only piles on the calories but also gives many people the mis-

FATS IN FOODS

Foods		Total fat in grams	Calories	% of cal from fat
Tuna	Chunk light in water, 3 oz (90 g), undrained	1.0	89	10
	Chunk light in oil, 3 oz (90 g), undrained	17.6	254	62
Chicken	Roasted light meat, no skin, 3½ oz (100 g)	4.5	171	24
	Fried battered, light with skin, 3½ oz (100 g)	15.3	274	50
Meat	Sirloin steak, lean only, broiled, 3 oz (90 g)	7.7	180	39
	Sirloin steak, lean & fat, broiled, 3 oz (90 g)	15.7	240	59
Milk	Skim milk, 1 cup (250 mL)	0.4	86	4
	Whole milk, 1 cup (250 mL)	8.1	150	49
Ice Cream	Vanilla-flavoured ice-milk, ½ cup (125 mL)	2.9	100	26
	Vanilla ice cream, ½ cup (125 mL)	17.9	260	62
Snacks	Pretzel twists, 1 oz (30 g)	0.9	110	7
	Potato chips, 1 oz (30 g)	11.7	160	66

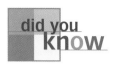

More than half the calories that people take in are burned up in basal metabolism—the energy we expend to stay alive.

Many people aren't aware that they need fewer calories as they get older. Not only does their metabolism slow down but they also tend to become less active.

So maintaining a healthy weight as you get older may require trimming your calorie intake.

The Japanese government suggests eating at least 30 different foods a day. By eating many different kinds of foods, it's almost certain that you will get a wide variety of nutrients. And most people can't overdo it on any one kind of food when they have 29 other kinds to fit into their diets.

taken idea that consuming the recommended five to nine servings of fruit and vegetables is hard to do. But actually, one serving of fruit is just a half cup—the size of the individual packs of applesauce or fruit salad that moms put into lunch boxes for their first-graders.

Diet Therapy for Arthritis: Does it Work?

The notion that some foods can make arthritis worse while others might ease its symptoms is both intriguing and controversial. Until recently, most experts were skeptical about diet therapy's role in arthritis care.

But studies over the past few years have shown that some dietary interventions may be useful, particularly for patients with inflammatory forms of arthritis such as RA. Here's a rundown of the main ways that diet has been used to treat arthritis—and what the evidence shows.

Avoidance Diets

These are based on the idea that certain foods are the aggressors when it comes to arthritis. By subtracting the offending foods from your diet, proponents claim, people with arthritis will experience significant improvements in their symptoms.

The anti-nightshade diet. Probably the best known avoidance diet, it's based on the idea that the "nightshade" family of foods—tomatoes, potatoes, eggplant, and peppers—contain chemicals that promote inflammation, increase pain and interfere with the repair of damaged joints.

The "nightshade theory" was proposed by horticulturist Norman Childers, who knew that tomatoes and other nightshades were once considered poisonous—

WHERE THE VITAMINS LIVE

Now that you know what anitoxidant vitamins can help your arthritis, where are you going to get them? Here is a guide to what foods contain which nutrients:

Beta carotene Yellow-orange fruits and vegetables such as apricots, sweet potatoes, pumpkin, carrots, cantaloupe, mangoes, papaya, peaches, and winter squash, as well as dark green leafy vegetables such as broccoli, spinach, collard greens, parsley and other leafy greens.

Vitamin C Cantaloupe, grapefruit, papaya, kiwi, oranges, mangoes, raspberries, pineapples, bananas, strawberries, tomatoes, and fresh vegetables such as Brussels sprouts, collard greens, cabbage, asparagus, broccoli, potatoes and red peppers.

Vitamin E Sunflower and safflower oils, sunflower seeds, wheat germ, nuts, avocados, peaches, whole-grain breads and cereals, spinach, broccoli, asparagus, dried prunes and peanut butter

and noticed that they seemed to worsen his arthritis. He carried out an uncontrolled study in which more than 5,000 arthritis patients were asked to avoid nightshade foods for seven years; nearly three-quarters of the patients said their pain and disability gradually improved.

The bottom line. The nightshade-free diet has never been studied in a scientifically rigorous way, though some rheumatologists have reported that a few of their patients improved after nightshades were removed from their diets. It can't hurt to try the diet (provided you don't make radical dietary changes that could interfere with nutrition), but don't expect much from it.

The Dong diet. Named for Collin Dong, the physician who devised it for his own arthritis, this diet is patterned

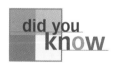

Nightshades come from the plant genus Solanum and include more than 1,700 herbs, shrubs and trees; including eggplant, bell peppers, potatoes and tomatoes. Although there are many claims that removing nightshades from your diet will cure arthritis, no scientific proof has yet been offered.

after one that many Chinese have followed for centuries. It imposes much broader food restrictions than the anti-nightshade diet. Arthritis patients are urged to eat vegetables but to eliminate red meat, fruit, dairy, herbs, alcohol, additives and preservatives.

In a 1983 study, some arthritis patients were placed on the Dong diet while others consumed a diet allowing for a variety of foods. No significant differences were noted, with about half the people in each group reporting that they felt better.

The bottom line. No scientific evidence supports the Dong diet, which could actually harm people with arthritis: The diet excludes joint-healthy fruit; and it bans dairy products, the main dietary source of the calcium and vitamin D needed to maintain bones and assist in cartilage formation.

Anti-Allergic Diets: They Caused a Reaction?

Many arthritis patients are convinced that some foods—particularly milk products, corn and cereals—not only aggravate their arthritis, but can actually trigger symptoms immediately, much as people with asthma may start coughing after inhaling pollen or other substances to which they're allergic.

Some people have genuine food allergies, in which a food protein prompts the immune system to produce antibodies against that protein, which is known as an antigen. Antibody combines with antigen to form antigen-antibody "complexes." Proponents of the allergy-arthritis notion contend that these antigen-antibody complexes could conceivably irritate the joints or even attack the joints' synovial lining.

Experts now believe that food sensitivities such as allergies may be involved in some cases of rheumatoid and other types of inflammatory arthritis. But the actual proportion of patients affected appears to be small—perhaps five percent or fewer. Consider the results of one study that involved 159 patients with RA, 52 of whom claimed that food aggravated their symptoms. Actual testing of all the patients failed to detect a single case of food intolerance.

Diets That Put Out the Fire?

Inflammation is the body's response to tissue damage or overuse of a diseased joint. Researchers have found that fatty acids may mitigate the inflammation response in certain types of arthritis, as can certain chemicals found in teas.

Fishing for Relief

Studies of Greenland Inuit led to interest in the anti-arthritic properties of fish. Although they lived mainly on fatty fish, these Inuit were found to have remarkably low levels of heart disease and RA. The beneficial effects of these cold-water fish were attributed to the omega-3 fatty acids that are plentiful in fish oil.

Researchers now know that a diet high in fish changes the lipids that make up cell membranes in the body, and this change reduces the level of inflammatory chemicals called cytokines.

FAT CONTENT OF SELECTED SEAFOOD

Foods (3 oz/85 grams)	Omega-3 fatty acids (g)	Saturated fat (g)	Total fat (g)	Calories
Atlantic salmon	1.9	1.1	6.9	155
Herring	1.8	2.2	9.8	172
Whitefish	1.6	1.0	6.4	146
Bluefin tuna	1.3	1.4	5.3	156
Sardines, canned, in oil	1.3	1.3	9.7	177
Mackerel	1.1	3.6	15.2	223
Rainbow trout	1.0	1.4	5.0	128

Several studies have shown fish-oil supplements may offer modest benefits for patients with RA inflammation. But it isn't known yet whether fish-oil supplements will benefit people with osteoarthritis—which typically doesn't involve inflammation.

Even if fish or fish-oil supplements don't help to ease your arthritis symptoms, consuming more fish makes a lot of sense. Studies show that people who eat fish regularly can gain some important health benefits.

➡ BONING UP: Eicosapentaenoic acid (EPA), best known of the omega-3 fatty acids, is found in marine plants and fish. EPA is actually made by algae, plankton and seaweed, which are then eaten by certain fish.

A study of American men found that those eating the most fish were about 40 percent less likely to die from a heart attack or clot-caused stroke over a six- to eight-year period than men who consumed the least fish. Also, researchers have found that the omega-3s in fatty fish are important for vision, nerve and immune function, and possibly for protection against some cancers.

The bottom line. All fish contain some omega-3 fatty acids. But to maximize your intake, choose oily cold-water fish such as salmon, tuna and mackerel (see table, page 210). Eating cold-water fish two or three times a week should help your overall health and could be of some help for your arthritis.

Sip Your Arthritis Symptoms Away?

If you have arthritis or just want to improve your general health, take a cue from the English and the Asians and have a spot of tea. Tea is rich in flavonoids, a class of phytochemicals known for its antioxidant abilities. Some studies have shown that regular tea drinkers are up to 50 percent less likely to develop certain types of cancer than non-tea drinkers, while other studies have found that regular tea drinkers have a lower risk of stroke and heart disease. And as noted earlier in this chapter, evidence suggests that diets rich in antioxidants can help keep osteoarthritis from worsening.

The green light to green tea. Both black and green teas are good sources of flavonoids. But now there is reason to believe that green tea may be particularly useful against rheumatoid arthritis, thanks to a different class of phytochemicals known as polyphenols, present in abundant amounts in green tea.

Researchers at Case Western Reserve University School of Medicine in Cleveland extracted polyphenols from green tea and added them to drinking water fed to young mice. Another group of mice received water without polyphenols. After all the mice were injected with a chemical that usually triggers a disease resembling RA, the mice who had consumed the polyphenols were much less likely to develop RA, and the cases that did occur were milder. Fewer than half the polyphenol-drinking mice even developed RA, compared with 94 percent of those drinking plain water.

The bottom line. Try drinking three or four cups of green tea daily without milk to see if it reduces inflammation. Note: Green tea does contain caffeine (about 40 mg a cup), so you may want to cut back on other sources of caffeine, such as coffee.

Try out these six key weight-loss tactics.

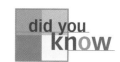

Letting green tea steep more than five minutes can cause the beneficial substances to lose their potency. Use one teaspoon of green tea leaves per cup of very hot (not boiling) water.

THE SIX Key Tactics for Weight Loss

Some people need a rigorous, clearly defined program to keep them on the weight-loss path. Others just need a nudge in the right direction. For those in the latter group, the following six tactics will give you the everyday secrets you need to start losing weight now.

Tactic 1: Cut Fat

Official recommendations limit fat to 30 percent of your total calorie intake (with carbs at 55 percent and protein at 15 percent) because fat contains twice the calories of the other nutrients. So cutting back on fatty fare goes further toward lightening your load than cutting the same amount of carbohydrate. But the kind of fat you eat is important as well. *Saturated* fat is most closely tied with cardiovascular risks.

Saturated fats are solid at room temperature, like butter, some cheeses and the fat on meats. These fats should account for no more than 10 percent of your total calories.

Omega-3s, and the monounsaturated fats in oils like canola, can actually be good for you. So, cut total fat to avoid extra calories, and switch to healthier fats for more arthritis-fighting nutrients. The Arthritis Foundation recommends trading corn, safflower and sunflower oils for olive, canola and flaxseed oils, and keeping your daily meat and poultry intake to an amount roughly equal to a deck of cards. Other suggestions:

- **Get milk.** Drink an extra glass of nonfat milk a day: Studies suggest that getting more calcium while cutting calories helps people lose more weight than dieting alone. Calcium intake is linked with less body fat and less weight gain in midlife. And getting protein from milk or other sources can help you feel full on less food.

- **De-blubber the broth.** Skim fat from soups by throwing a few ice cubes into the pot: The fat will coagulate and cling to the ice after sitting a few minutes and come out of the broth when you take out the cubes.

- **Use your napkin.** Most fats are liquid when heated, so they can be blotted off with a napkin. Next time you get pizza, sop up the oil on top. With meats, sop up the juices when serving. When browning ground beef, pour out the oil and rub the meat down with a paper towel.

- **Cut the butter.** Yes, butter is delicious, but it is also almost pure saturated fat. Find alternatives.

Dip breads in olive oil or spread with jam rather than buttering. Use salsa on baked potatoes. Experiment with low-fat or no-fat cream cheese spreads and herbs.

Tactic 2: Pare Portions

One reason for all these calories is that these days, portions are huge. Studies find that hamburgers and fries (two notorious examples) are generally offered in serving sizes two to five times larger than the appropriate meal size. Not that we tend to care: Researchers find we usually clean our plates no matter how high they're piled, even if we already feel satisfied. These portions are one likely reason North Americans continue getting fatter even as the percentage of our total calories from fat has gone down in recent years. But portions are simple to control because it's easier to count cookies than calories. To begin with, eat out less: Restaurant portions are larger than most people serve at home, and you're more likely to eat fatty food when eating out. Also check food labels when shopping for home: Packages list the calories in specific portion sizes—which may be smaller than you think. Other suggestions:

- **Eat healthy.** Health Canada's website has a whole section devoted to using Canada's Food Guide to improve your health and weight. Check it out at **www.hc-sc.gc.ca/fn-an/food-guide-aliment/index_e.html**.

- **Picture portions.** Use familiar objects to picture how much you should eat of a food before you pick up your fork or spoon. For example, a half-cup (125 mL) of low-fat granola is about the size of your fist. The same amount of low-fat vanilla ice cream equals half an orange, size-wise. And a serving of meat, chicken or fish should be the size of a deck of cards.

- **Consider the four-quarters rule.** The perfect plate has a starch in one quarter, a protein in another, and vegetables in the remaining half.

- **Use a smaller dish.** Sounds ridiculous, but it works. Obviously, you can't put as much food on a salad plate. But you're also just not inclined to eat as quickly if your plate will be empty in 45 seconds.

● **Keep the seconds far away.** If you put the extra chicken or mashed potatoes on the table, all you have to do is reach over to get to them. If they are back in the kitchen, or already put away, you'll be less inclined to keep gobbling food.

● **Have raw vegetables at every meal.** Raw cucumbers, tomatoes, peppers and celery have few calories and lots of nutrients. A plate in the middle of the table almost always gets eaten up, cutting down appetite for the more calorie-dense meat or starch courses.

● **Start your meal with soup.** Studies show that a bowl of soup at the start of the meal reduces overall meal consumption. Consommés and brothy vegetable soups are best, since they are lowest in calories and highest in nutrients.

● **Manage your fork.** After every bite, put your fork down. Don't pick it up until you have thoroughly chewed and swallowed. The goal is both to slow down your eating and to eat less. Remember: Your body digests for 20 minutes before sending signals to your brain that you are no longer hungry.

● **Have a snack.** Forget the idea that you'll eat less if you quit noshing between meals—the opposite is true. While you don't want to overeat, occasional snacking on low-calorie foods helps you feel satisfied and less prone to overdoing it when you finally sit down to a meal. Feeding small amounts of food into your system also keeps your energy up throughout the day and doesn't overload your digestive system at mealtime. Some ideal snacks: carrot or zucchini sticks with salsa, pretzels with low-sodium vegetable juice and air-popped popcorn without butter. Get in the habit of two-to-three 100-calorie snacks per day.

Tactic 3: Sidestep Sugars

Avoiding sugar has always meant limiting sweets and soft drinks because they contain too many empty calories and too few nutrients. But now concerns about sugar have broadened to include other types of simple carbohydrates, especially refined starches like white bread and potatoes. Controversial low-carb diets have long held that excess carbohydrates are the true cause of weight gain. And there may be something to it: In one study, published in *The New England Journal of Medicine,* people on a low-carb diet that included omega-3 fatty acids lost three times more weight than people on a low-fat diet over a period of six months.

The long-term effects of such diets aren't well studied and it remains to be seen whether they're better at keeping weight off over time. "At this point, nobody can justify a dogmatic stance on where calories should come from," says Murray. But many researchers endorse the idea of avoiding simple starches and sugars, which may cause chemical changes in the body that lead to weight gain, in favour of whole grains, healthy fats and lots of vegetables. Here are everyday ways to do so:

● **Rethink breakfast.** Pancakes, muffins, bagels, doughnuts—they're all big blasts of simple carbohydrates. Here's the perfect breakfast: one serving of fruit, one serving of dairy and one serving of a complex carb. For dairy: low-fat milk or yogourt. For the carbohydrate: a slice of whole-wheat toast or a multigrain breakfast bar. Fruit is your choice.

● **Rethink dessert.** The old line is that you only get dessert if you clean your plate. Hmmm… sounds like a formula for obesity! Desserts are often filled with white flour, sugar, butter and other empty calories. Instead, clean your plate so you *won't* want dessert. Make dessert one of your two or three 100-calorie snacks for the day. Or skip an immediate dessert: wait an hour or two after supper, and if you are hungry, opt for a fistful of fresh strawberries or an orange.

● **Break the code.** When grocery shopping, check labels for terms such as fructose, sucrose and dextrose—all of which indicate there's sugar in the food. And don't be fooled by terms like "no added sugar," which can be used to disguise high amounts of natural sugar.

● **Forgo fructose.** Watch out for corn syrup, a sweetener that's loaded into soft drinks and many processed foods. And it's not just the empty calories: Studies suggest corn syrup fails to trigger hormones that regulate body weight and appetite.

● **Junk juices.** Replace fruit drinks, sports drinks and pop with plain or sparkling water and add a wedge of lemon for flavour: drinking just one less sweet drink a day will lower your calorie tally enough to keep off an extra 10 pounds in a year.

● **Gravitate to whole-grain.** Eat whole-grain foods, such as whole-wheat bread—they contain more complex carbohydrates than foods made with refined flour, like white bread. Complex carbs are absorbed slowly by the body and are thought to pose less of a weight gain risk than foods made from refined-flour.

● **Order it brown.** Some Asian restaurants now give you the option of brown rice or white rice. Choose brown rice: It is the whole-grain version that is much healthier and more filling than white.

Tactic 4: Tame Your Appetite

We tend to think appetite is the equivalent of the "empty" gauge on a dashboard: It lets you know you're low on fuel, so you stop to fill up. But that's actually a better way of describing the mechanisms of hunger, which are different from those of appetite. Hunger is a biological drive to make sure you eat enough, while appetite is a complex mix of body chemistry, habit, social behaviour and psychology that's notoriously difficult to manage. But the task isn't impossible, especially as researchers and therapists devote more attention to understanding the power of appetite and how to subdue it.

● **Ask yourself why.** For many, meals aren't the reason we gain weight—it's all the nibbling and snacking we do in between. Experts point out that much of this kind of eating has nothing to do with hunger. Rather, it's boredom, stress or a learned habit independent of appetite (3:30 p.m.—time to get a snack at the vending machine!). There's a simple antidote: Ask yourself why you are putting food in your mouth. If it's not because of hunger, stop.

● **Find alternatives.** So if so much eating is about boredom, stress or habit, what to do when you are bored, stressed or in need of a ritual? Easy: Take a walk. Put on music. Do a stretch routine. Go outside. Phone a friend. Read a favourite

magazine. Knit—whatever gives you pleasure and relaxation. If you can create a new routine to deal with everyday challenges that doesn't involve food, you will make major strides toward losing weight.

● **Turn on the lights.** Wandering into the kitchen at night? Flip on the light. Research at the University of California, Irvine, suggests that you feel in the spotlight when you're brightly illuminated. The sense of being on display will make you less likely to go on an ice cream bender.

● **Go to the candle store.** Next time you get a craving, light a scented candle: Studies suggest that certain aromas can take the edge off your appetite. The smells that work best include green apple, peppermint and banana.

● **Pressure your appetite.** You won't find this in the National Library of Medicine, but when you feel weak-willed against your appetite, try pinching the small area of cartilage where your jaws hinge just below the ears, which some acupuncturists claim is an appetite control point. Hold for about half a minute.

● **Eat power pleasers.** To eat less at meals and snack time, choose foods with a high satiety index—meaning they're more satisfying than other foods. Surprisingly, even though fatty foods fill you up and provide pleasure, they're not high scorers on the satiety scale because we tend to want more of them. Among the most satisfying foods: Popcorn, jellybeans, potatoes, brown pasta, baked beans, grapes and oranges.

Tactic 5: Make Small Lifestyle Adjustments

Again, lasting weight loss is more about small living and eating adjustments than it is following an intense short-term program that changes all aspects of your diet. The latter might deliver dramatic losses in the short term, but once the diet is over... Here are some tips that can give your permanent weight-loss efforts the edge you need to succeed:

● **Forget weight.** Too many people focus on pounds when it comes to measuring weight loss. Instead, focus on your energy level, how your joints are feeling, how your clothes are fitting and how you look in the mirror. Sure, your weight is the clearest measurement of your progress, but your health and happiness are a better scale. If your joints are telling you your weight-loss efforts are helping, then there's no better measurement.

● **Develop movement habits.** Research shows that people who fidget burn 500 or more extra calories in a day. All extra movements burn calories, so develop movement habits. Examples: Stand when on the phone; leave the room during TV commercials; walk 10 minutes after supper; tap your foot to music. Develop one or two such habits and you'll burn many more calories.

● **Drink water.** You've heard the health benefits of water many times, so do it: Get a water bottle or travel mug, fill it up after breakfast and keep it with you. Refill, refill, refill. At the end of the day, wash it out for tomorrow.

● **Entertain your mouth.** Sometimes all it takes to halt the snacking is a piece of gum, a slow-to-dissolve piece of candy or a toothpick. While society looks down on overt mouth habits, if you can be subtle, there's nothing wrong with an hour-long engagement with a piece of sugarless gum.

● **Shop the perimeter.** At the grocery store, the healthy produce, meats, seafood, dairy and bakery are usually around the perimeter. Cookies, chips, canned or boxed foods, and ice cream are in the aisles. Shop only along the store perimeter, delving once a month into the aisles for staples.

● **Spice up your meals.** Add zest to food with cayenne, jalapeños, ginger, Tabasco sauce and mustard. Studies find that the thermogenic properties of zingier foods boost your metabolism's fat-burning ability by as much as 25 percent.

● **Sleep better.** It sounds like quackery, but you really can encourage weight loss by sleeping. Research into sleep and hormone function finds that your metabolism rises and you burn calories more efficiently when you're well rested.

● **Nix Nickelodeon.** Watching TV with the kids? Tune out the commercials. Children's programming contains an average of 2,800 calories per hour, according to researchers at the University of California, Davis. And seeing less food on the tube translates to less junk in the pantry.

● **Top your tank before exercise.** Have a well-balanced carbohydrate/protein snack (half an apple with peanut butter or crackers with cheese) an hour before a workout. The carbs will keep your energy up and the protein will slow your digestion, giving you stamina you need.

● **Skip the wine.** If you sip a glass of wine or beer with meals, think about a prohibition diet. The drink isn't bad per se, but your body tends to prioritize processing alcohol, making calories from food more likely to be stored as fat, according to researchers at Pennsylvania State University.

● **Do the ring test.** Even if you don't have high blood pressure, try this test: Slip a ring onto your finger. Now eat salty food, wait a few hours and try to take the ring off. If sliding the ring is more difficult, you're probably someone for whom salt causes bloat—potentially grounds for extra pounds, according to researchers at the University of Maryland. Check food labels for sodium.

Tactic 6: Eat Well—and Enjoy Eating!

When it comes to managing arthritis, fixing a good meal is no different from choosing the right medicine, enjoying exercise and keeping a positive attitude. All are integral to the everyday arthritis solution.

Developing a love of food that tastes good *and* is good for you can take practice and a guiding hand. The following recipes are rich in the nutrients that are so important to joint health, modest in calories and as easy to prepare as they are yummy. While these meals won't give you *instantaneous* arthritis relief, a consistent diet of this type can lead to significant joint improvement.

RECIPES FOR BEATING ARTHRITIS

Breakfast

Asparagus & Red Pepper Frittata, 217

Blueberry & Cranberry Granola, 217

Whole-Wheat Breakfast Muffins, 218

Eggs in Tortilla Flowers, 218

Orange-Banana Breakfast Smoothie, 219

Strawberry-Yogourt Smoothie, 219

Soups

Lemony Lentil Soup, 220

Black Bean Soup, 220

Chunky Beet, Potato & Beef Soup, 221

Creamy Cabbage & Carrot Soup, 221

Portuguese Kale Soup, 222

Sweet Corn Chowder, 222

Salads

Arugula Salad with Spicy Vinaigrette, 223

Bread Salad with Roasted Peppers, 223

Crab & Grapefruit Salad, 224

Cold Tuna & Vegetable Salad, 224

Spinach Salad with Chickpeas, 225

Smoked Turkey & Melon Salad, 226

Warm Snow Pea Salad with Mushrooms & Goat Cheese, 226

Meat

Grilled Steak & Vegetables, 227

Italian Beef & Broccoli Sauté, 227

Spicy Lamb Stew with Couscous, 228

Lamb Curry, 229

Mediterranean Lamb Roast & Potatoes, 229

Spinach-Stuffed Meat Loaf, 230

Beef & Turkey Chili, 230

Poultry

Chicken Stew with Balsamic Vinegar, 231

Grilled Chicken with Herbs, 231

Spicy Asian Chicken Braised with Mushrooms, 232

Pesto Chicken on Focaccia, 232

Poached Chicken, 233

Sesame Chicken Salad, 233

Thai Chicken Stew, 234

Jamaican Jerked Chicken Salad, 234

Turkey Quesadillas, 236

Fish

Salmon Steaks Mexican-Style, 236

Broiled Herb-Rubbed Salmon, 237

Summer Salmon & Asparagus, 237

Walnut-Crusted Snapper, 238

Garlic, Tomato & Anchovy Toasts, 238

Grilled Halibut Steaks with Tomato & Red Pepper Salsa, 239

Asian Stuffed Shrimp Salad, 239

French Shrimp Stew, 240

Broiled Salmon with Avocado-Mango Salsa, 240

Pasta, Beans & Grains

Penne with Sugar Snaps & Smoked Salmon, 242

Creole-Style Beans, 242

Risotto with Spring Vegetables, 243

Tex-Mex Turkey, Corn & Barley Casserole, 243

Herbed Polenta, 244

Vegetables

Apricot-Maple Acorn Squash, 244

Orange-Glazed Carrots, 244

Roasted New Potatoes, 245

Sweet Roasted Squash with Shallots, 245

Sweet Potato & Apple Bake, 245

Desserts

Pineapple Foster, 246

Caramelized Orange Compote, 246

Berry Sorbet, 247

Chocolate-Hazelnut Cheesecake, 247

Three Berry Fool, 248

Ginger Pancake with Banana-Walnut Topping, 248

Mixed Berry Tart, 250

Asparagus & Red Pepper Frittata

Asparagus and olive oil add vitamin E to this lovely brunch dish; the red bell pepper adds vitamin C, and the cheese supplies calcium. All make this a powerhouse anti-arthritis recipe.

PREPARATION TIME: 10 MINUTES

COOKING TIME: 20 MINUTES • SERVES 4

½ lb (250 g) asparagus, trimmed and cut into ½-in. (1-cm) lengths
red bell pepper, cut into ½-in. (1-cm) squares
3 eggs
4 egg whites
2 tsp (10 mL) flour
½ cup (125 mL) grated Parmesan cheese
½ tsp (2 mL) salt
¼ tsp (1 mL) black pepper
2 tsp (10 mL) olive oil
1 tsp (5 mL) unsalted butter

1. In medium pot of boiling water, cook asparagus and bell pepper for 2 minutes to blanch; drain well.

2. In medium bowl, whisk together whole eggs and egg whites. Whisk in flour until well combined. Whisk in Parmesan cheese, salt and black pepper. Stir in asparagus and bell pepper.

3. In 10-in. (25-cm) cast-iron or other broiler-proof skillet, heat oil and butter over low heat until butter has melted. Pour in egg mixture and cook without stirring for 15 minutes or until eggs are set around the edges and almost set in centre. Meanwhile, preheat broiler.

4. Broil frittata 6 in. (15 cm) from heat for 1 to 2 minutes or until top is just set. Cut into wedges and serve hot, warm, or at room temperature.

Calories: 170, fat: 10 g, saturated fat: 4 g, sodium: 530 mg, carbohydrate: 6 g, protein: 15 g.

Blueberry & Cranberry Granola

This delicious toasted cereal is made from a mix of vitamin E-rich grains, nuts and seeds, and vitamin C-rich berries. Canola oil adds omega-3 fatty acids. Stirring maple syrup and orange juice into the granola helps to keep the oil content down, making this version much lower in calories than most "crunchy" cereals you buy.

PREPARATION TIME: 40-50 MINUTES, PLUS COOLING

MAKES ABOUT 8 SERVINGS

2 ¾ cups (675 mL) oatmeal
½ cup (125 mL) wheat germ
7 tbsp (110 mL) millet flakes
2 tbsp (25 mL) sunflower seeds
2 tbsp (25 mL) slivered almonds
1 tbsp (15 mL) sesame seeds
½ cup (125 mL) dried blueberries
½ cup (125 mL) dried cranberries
1 tbsp (15 mL) soft light brown sugar
2 tbsp (25 mL) maple syrup
2 tbsp (25 mL) canola oil
2 tbsp (25 mL) orange juice

1. Preheat oven to 325°F (160°C). In large bowl, combine oats, wheat germ, millet flakes, sunflower seeds, almonds, sesame seeds, dried berries, and sugar. Stir until well mixed.

2. In measuring cup, whisk together maple syrup, oil and orange juice. Pour mixture slowly into dry ingredients, stirring until liquid is evenly distributed and coats everything lightly.

3. In nonstick roasting pan, spread out mixture evenly. Bake until slightly crisp and lightly brown, 30 to 40 minutes, stirring every 10 minutes to encourage even browning.

4. Remove roasting pan from oven and leave granola to cool. Store in airtight container up to 2 weeks. Serve with plain yogourt, milk or fruit juice.

Calories: 250, fat: 7 g, saturated fat: 1 g, sodium: 5 mg, carbohydrate: 45 g, protein: 6 g.

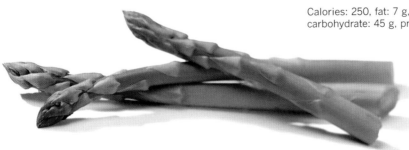

Whole-Wheat Breakfast Muffins

Muffins are always welcome at breakfast; these have low-fat yogourt for calcium, wheat germ for vitamin E, canola oil for omega-3 fatty acids, and orange juice and zest for vitamin C.

PREPARATION TIME: 15 MINUTES

COOKING TIME: 15-20 MINUTES • MAKES 12 MUFFINS

2/3 cup (150 mL) whole-wheat flour
3/4 cup (175 mL) plus 2 tbsp (25 mL)
    all-purpose flour
2 tsp (10 mL) baking soda
1 pinch (0.2 mL) salt
1/4 tsp (1 mL) cinnamon
1/4 cup (50 mL) packed dark brown sugar
5 tbsp (75 mL) wheat germ
1 cup (250 mL) packed raisins
1 cup (250 mL) plain low-fat yogourt
4 tbsp (60 mL) canola oil
1 large egg
Grated zest of 1/2 orange
3 tbsp (45 mL) orange juice

1. Preheat oven to 400°F (200°C). Grease 12-cup muffin pan.

2. Sift whole-wheat and all-purpose flours, baking soda, salt and cinnamon into large bowl, tipping in any bran left in the sieve. Stir in sugar, wheat germ and raisins, and make a well in the middle.

3. In small bowl, lightly whisk together yogourt, oil, egg, orange zest and juice. Pour liquid ingredients into well in flour mixture and stir together just enough to moisten dry ingredients. Don't beat or overmix.

4. Spoon batter into muffin pan, filling each cup 2/3 full. Bake until muffins are just firm to the touch, 15 to 20 minutes. Leave muffins to cool in tray 2 to 3 minutes, then turn out onto wire rack. The muffins are best still warm from the oven. Leftover muffins can be cooled completely and stored in an airtight container up to 2 days.

Calories: 190, fat: 6 g, saturated fat: 1 g, sodium: 240 mg, carbohydrate: 20 g, protein: 5 g.

Eggs in Tortilla Flowers

Vitamin D from the eggs, vitamin C from the red pepper, and omega-3s from the canola oil make this a powerful starter for the day.

PREPARATION TIME: 15 MINUTES

COOKING TIME: 20 MINUTES • SERVES 4

Nonstick cooking spray
4 corn tortillas, 6 in. (15 cm) in diameter
2 tsp (10 mL) canola oil
6 large eggs
4 large egg whites
2 tbsp (25 mL) water
1/4 tsp (1 mL) black pepper, or to taste
1 large sweet red pepper, cored, seeded, and
    finely chopped (1 cup/250 mL)
4 oz (125 g) reduced-sodium ham, finely
    cubed
2 scallions, including tops, sliced
Salsa (optional topping)

1. Preheat oven to 325°F (160°C). On baking sheet, invert 4 small custard cups or ovenproof glasses and coat bottoms with nonstick cooking spray. Brush each tortilla with 1/4 tsp (1 mL) oil, then cut 8 evenly spaced 2-in. (5-cm) deep slits around the edge. Centre each tortilla, oiled side up, on top of a cup, letting cut edges drape down sides. Bake for 20 minutes or until crisp.

2. After tortillas have baked for 10 minutes, start eggs. In medium bowl, beat together eggs, egg whites, water and black pepper. In 10-in. (25-cm) nonstick skillet over moderately low heat, heat remaining oil. Add red pepper, ham and scallions. Cover and cook for 6 minutes or until softened.

3. Add egg mixture and cook, uncovered, 3 minutes more, scrambling eggs lightly until they are just set. Remove tortillas from the custard cups and invert them on 4 individual serving plates. They will have formed shallow, flowerlike cups. Fill each tortilla flower with egg mixture and serve immediately. Top with salsa if desired.

Calories: 270, fat: 13 g, saturated fat: 3 g, sodium: 460 mg, carbohydrate: 19 g, protein: 20 g.

Orange-Banana Breakfast Smoothie

Vitamin C from the orange juice and vitamin B_6 from the banana make this a most refreshing eye opener.

PREPARATION TIME: 5 MINUTES • SERVES 1

3/4 cup (175 mL) orange juice
1/2 cup (125 mL) sliced banana
2 tsp (10 mL) brown sugar
1/8 tsp (0.5 mL) almond extract.
2 ice cubes
1 mint sprig

1. In blender, combine orange juice, banana, sugar and almond extract.

2. Add ice cubes and blend until thick and smooth.

3. Garnish with mint sprig.

Calories: 190, fat: 0 g, saturated fat: 0 g, sodium: 0 mg, carbohydrate: 46 g, protein: 2 g.

Strawberry-Yogourt Smoothie

This refreshing drink provides a healthy start to the day, with its high vitamin C and calcium content and natural sweetness. Dilute it with extra orange juice if you want a thinner drink.

PREPARATION TIME: 5 MINUTES • SERVES 4

1 lb (500 g) ripe strawberries, hulled
Grated zest and juice of 1 large orange
2/3 cup (150 mL) plain low-fat yogourt
1 tbsp (15 mL) sugar, or to taste (optional)
4 small strawberries (optional)
4 small orange slices (optional)

1. Put strawberries into food processor or blender. Add zest, juice and yogourt. Purée, scraping down sides of container once or twice. Taste mixture and sweeten with sugar, if necessary.

2. Pour into glasses. If you like, decorate with small strawberries and slices of orange, both split so they sit on the rim of the glass.

Calories: 90, fat: 0 g, saturated fat: 0 g, sodium: 35 mg, carbohydrate: 17 g, protein: 3 g.

Lemony Lentil Soup

This sturdy winter soup has a delicious citrus overtone combined with the warm flavours of roasted spices. The lentils provide you with almost a day's requirement of folate as well as some vitamin B$_6$. The lemon juice gives you vitamin C.

PREPARATION TIME: 5 MINUTES

COOKING TIME: 35 MINUTES • SERVES 4

1 tbsp (15 mL) olive oil

3 cloves garlic, chopped coarsely

1 medium onion, chopped

1⅓ cup (325 mL) red lentils, rinsed and drained

4 cups (1 L) chicken or vegetable broth

1 tsp (5 mL) ground coriander

½ tsp (2 mL) ground cumin

Juice of 1 lemon

4 wafer-thin slices of lemon

1. In large heavy pot over medium heat, cook garlic and onions in oil until brown, 3 to 5 minutes. Add lentils and cook, stirring, 2 minutes. Stir in broth. Simmer soup, covered, until lentils are almost soft, 15 to 20 minutes.

2. In dry skillet set over high heat, toast coriander and cumin until aromatic, 1 to 2 minutes, then add to soup. Add lemon juice, lemon slices, and salt and pepper to taste, and simmer soup for 5 minutes before serving.

Calories: 280, fat: 5 g, saturated fat: 1 g, sodium: 130 mg, carbohydrate: 41 g, protein: 18 g.

Black Bean Soup

Black beans are high in folate and calcium; bell peppers and tomatoes are high in vitamin C. This soup is, therefore, as healthy as it is delicious.

PREPARATION TIME: 5 MINUTES

COOKING TIME: 7 MINUTES • SERVES 4

1 diced green bell pepper

2 sliced scallions

3 cloves minced garlic

2 tsp (10 mL) oil

1 can (19 oz/540 mL) black beans, rinsed and drained

1½ cups (375 mL) chicken broth

1 tsp (5 mL) each ground coriander and cumin

2 tbsp (25 mL) reduced-fat sour cream

¼ cup (50 mL) diced tomato

1. In pot, sauté bell pepper, scallions and garlic in oil until soft.

2. Add black beans, chicken broth, coriander and cumin. Simmer 5 minutes.

3. In blender or food processor, purée half the soup and return to pan; reheat soup. Top with sour cream and tomato.

Calories: 180, fat: 5 g, saturated fat: 1 g, sodium: 460 mg, carbohydrate: 24 g, protein: 10 g.

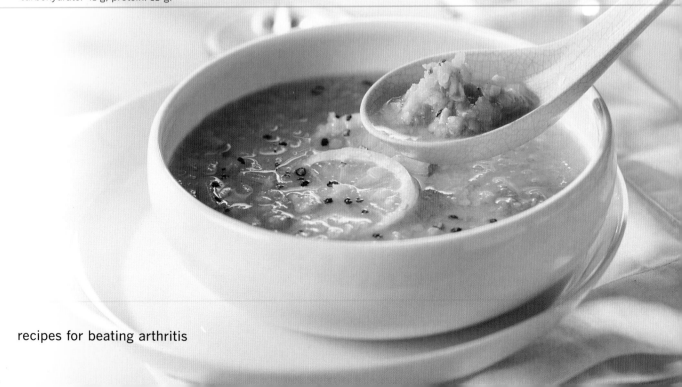

Chunky Beet, Potato & Beef Soup

Here's a healthy, hearty version of borscht, the famous Eastern European beet soup. The beets are full of folate and vitamin C, and the potatoes contribute vitamins C and B₆.

PREPARATION TIME: 30 MINUTES

COOKING TIME: 35 MINUTES • SERVES 4

2 tsp (10 mL) olive oil
6 scallions, thinly sliced
4 cloves garlic, minced
2½ lb (1.15 kg) fresh beets, peeled and cut into ½-in. (1-cm) cubes
¾ lb (375 g) all-purpose potatoes, peeled and cut into 1/2-in. (1-cm) cubes
2 carrots, thinly sliced
¼ cup (50 mL) red wine vinegar
4 teaspoons sugar
1 tsp (5 mL) salt
¼ tsp (1 mL) pepper
¾ lb (375 g) well-trimmed top round beef steak, cut into ¼-in. (0.6-cm) chunks
¼ cup (50 mL) reduced-fat sour cream

1. In large pot, heat oil over moderate heat. Add scallions and garlic, and sauté for 2 minutes or until scallions are tender.

2. Add beets, potatoes, carrots, vinegar, sugar, salt, pepper and 4½ cups (1.13 L) water. Bring to a boil, reduce to a simmer, cover, and cook for 15 minutes or until beets and potatoes are almost tender. Add beef and cook for 15 minutes or until just cooked through. Serve topped with a dollop of sour cream.

Calories: 440, fat: 8 g, saturated fat: 5 g, sodium: 760 mg, carbohydrate: 55 g, protein: 38 g.

Creamy Cabbage & Carrot Soup

You can make this soup with crinkly Savoy cabbage, which is rich in folate and vitamin C. The carrots and tomato paste add more vitamin C. The sour cream contributes calcium.

PREPARATION TIME: 15 MINUTES

COOKING TIME: 40 MINUTES • SERVES 4

1 tbsp (15 mL) olive oil
1 large onion, finely chopped
4 cloves garlic, minced
2 carrots, thinly sliced
8 cups (2 L) shredded green cabbage
2½ cups (625 mL) chicken broth
¾ cup (175 mL) snipped fresh dill
⅓ cup (75 mL) no-salt-added tomato paste
¾ tsp (4 mL) ground ginger
¼ tsp (1 mL) each salt and pepper
⅓ cup (75 mL) reduced-fat sour cream

1. In large Dutch oven or flameproof casserole, heat oil over moderate heat. Add onion and garlic, and sauté for 7 minutes or until the onion is soft. Add carrots and sauté for 5 minutes or until the carrots are crisp-tender.

2. Stir in cabbage, cover and cook, stirring occasionally, for 10 minutes or until cabbage is wilted.

3. Add broth, 2½ cups (625 mL) water, dill, tomato paste, ginger, salt, and pepper. Bring to a boil, reduce to a simmer, cover, and cook for 15 minutes or until cabbage is very tender. Stir sour cream into soup.

Calories: 180, fat: 9 g, saturated fat: 3 g, sodium: 810 mg, carbohydrate: 22 g, protein: 5 g.

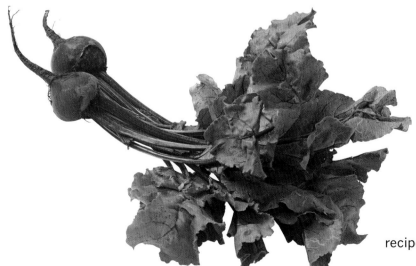

recipes for beating arthritis   221

Portuguese Kale Soup

Rich in calcium and vitamin C, kale tastes great teamed with sausage, potatoes (with their vitamin C and B₆), and kidney beans (good sources of folate and vitamin B₆).

PREPARATION TIME: 20 MINUTES • COOKING TIME:

45 MINUTES • MAKES SIX 1½-CUP (375-ML) SERVINGS

- 4 oz (125 g) spicy turkey sausage or Italian sausage
- 1½ oz (45 g) sliced pepperoni, slivered
- 1 large yellow onion, quartered and thinly sliced (1½ cups/375 mL)
- 1 medium stalk celery, coarsely chopped (½ cup/125 mL)
- 1 can (14 oz/398 mL) low-sodium chicken broth mixed with 6 cups (1.5 L) water
- 8 oz (250 g) kale, thick stems removed and leaves sliced (about 8 cups/2 L), or 2 packages (10 oz/300 g each) frozen kale, thawed and squeezed dry
- ½ tsp (2 mL) minced garlic
- 12 oz (375 g) red-skin potatoes, halved and sliced (2 cups)
- ½ tsp (2 mL) hot red pepper sauce, or to taste
- ¼ tsp (1 mL) salt, or to taste
- 1½ cups (375 mL) cooked red kidney beans

1. Remove casings from sausage and discard; crumble meat. In stockpot or 5-qt (5-L) Dutch oven over moderately low heat, cook sausage, stirring, for 4 minutes. Add pepperoni and cook 2 minutes more or until fat is rendered. Drain sausage and pepperoni on paper towels. Pour out all but 1 tsp (15 mL) fat from stockpot and discard.

2. Add onion and celery to stockpot and cook over low heat, covered, stirring occasionally, 8 minutes or until softened. Return sausage to stockpot and add stock, kale and garlic. Bring to a simmer, cover, and cook 10 minutes.

3. Stir in potatoes, red pepper sauce and salt. Simmer, covered, 20 minutes more or until potatoes and kale are tender. Add beans and cook just until heated through.

Calories: 229, fat: 7 g, saturated fat: 2 g, sodium: 498 mg, carbohydrate: 30 g, protein: 13 g.

Sweet Corn Chowder

Corn is high in folate, the other vegetables add vitamin C, and the milk adds calcium to this all-time favorite soup that is actually good for you!

PREPARATION TIME: 20 MINUTES

COOKING TIME: 45 MINUTES • MAKES 11 CUPS (2.6 L)

- 2 oz (60 g) reduced-sodium bacon, coarsely chopped
- 2 large onions, diced
- 2 large carrots, diced
- 2 stalks celery, diced
- 12 oz (375 g) all-purpose potatoes, peeled and diced
- 6 cups (1.5 L) chicken stock
- 2 cups (500 mL) fresh or frozen corn kernels
- 2 cups (500 mL) 1% low-fat milk
- ⅛ tsp (0.5 mL) each salt and pepper
- Cayenne pepper

1. In 4-qt (4-L) pot over moderate heat, cook bacon until browned and fat rendered, about 4 minutes. Remove bacon with slotted spoon and reserve for garnish.

2. Add onions, carrots and celery to pot and sauté until softened, about 5 minutes.

3. Stir in potatoes with chicken stock and bring to boil. Simmer soup, partially covered, stirring occasionally, until vegetables are tender, about 10 minutes.

4. Add corn kernels and return soup to boil. Simmer, uncovered, about 5 minutes longer.

5. Remove from heat and, using a ladle or slotted spoon, transfer about 2½ cups (635 mL) of vegetables to a blender or food processor. Purée until smooth.

6. Add purée and milk to pot and simmer about 3 minutes. Season with salt, pepper and a pinch of cayenne. Serve garnished with bacon.

Per cup: Calories: 88, fat: 3 g, saturated fat: 1 g, sodium: 87 mg, carbohydrate: 14 g, protein: 4 g.

Arugula Salad with Spicy Vinaigrette

This tart and refreshing side dish or appetizer has lots of vitamin C from the orange and its juice, the tomatoes, and even the greens. The arugula is also very high in calcium.

PREPARATION TIME: 25 MINUTES • SERVES 4

½ cup (125 mL) orange juice
2 tbsp (25 mL) red wine vinegar
2 tsp (10 mL) jalapeño pepper sauce
1 tsp (5 mL) olive oil
½ tsp (2 mL) salt
¼ tsp (1 mL) sugar
⅛ tsp (0.5 mL) pepper
8 cups (2 L) arugula leaves
2 cups (500 mL) torn romaine lettuce
1 cup (250 mL) yellow and/or red cherry tomatoes, halved
1 navel orange, peeled and sliced into half-rounds
6 oil-cured black olives, slivered
½ small red onion, thinly sliced

1. In small bowl, whisk together orange juice, vinegar, jalapeño pepper sauce, oil, salt, sugar and pepper.

2. In salad bowl, combine arugula, lettuce, tomatoes, orange, olives and onion. Add dressing, tossing to coat well. Serve immediately.

Calories: 70, fat: 2 g, saturated fat: 0 g, sodium: 310 mg, carbohydrate: 13 g, protein: 3 g.

Bread Salad with Roasted Peppers

Red peppers have far more vitamin C than green peppers, making this a power dish for people with arthritis.

PREPARATION TIME: 15 MINUTES

COOKING TIME: 20 MINUTES • SERVES 4

4 large red bell peppers, cored and cut into flat panels
2 tbsp (25 mL) balsamic vinegar
1 tbsp (15 mL) olive oil
2 cups (500 mL) Italian or French bread cubes (1 in./2.5 cm)
3 large tomatos, diced
1½ cups (375 mL) diced cucumber
3 oz (85 g) feta cheese, crumbled
¼ cup (50 mL) coarsely chopped kalamata or other brine-cured olives

1. Preheat broiler. Place peppers, skin side up, on rack of broiling pan and broil 4 in. (10 cm) from heat for 12 minutes or until skin is blackened. Remove from broiler and allow to cool in brown paper bag. Peel cooled peppers and cut into 2-in. (5 cm) wide strips.

2. In medium bowl, combine vinegar and oil. Add peppers and toss well. Refrigerate for at least 1 hour.

3. Preheat oven to 375°F (190°C). Spread bread cubes on baking sheet and bake, tossing occasionally, for 7 minutes or until lightly crisped, but not browned.

4. In large salad bowl, combine peppers and their marinade with toasted bread, tomato, cucumber, feta and olives, tossing well. Serve at room temperature or chilled.

Calories: 340, fat: 13 g, saturated fat: 4 g, sodium: 750 mg, carbohydrate: 46 g, protein: 11 g.

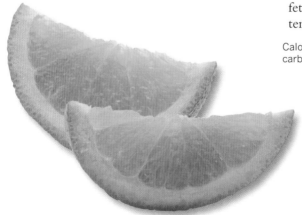

recipes for beating arthritis   **223**

Crab & Grapefruit Salad

A summer treat that provides omega-3 fatty acids from the crab as well as lots of vitamin C from the grapefruit and calcium from the greens.

PREPARATION TIME: 25 MINUTES • SERVES 4

4 grapefruits
2 tbsp (25 mL) light mayonnaise
1 tbsp (15 mL) finely chopped mango
  chutney
2 tsp (10 mL) Dijon mustard
1 tsp (5 mL) sesame oil
1/4 tsp (1 mL) each salt and pepper
3/4 lb (375 g) lump crabmeat, picked over to
  remove any cartilage
2 cups (500 mL) watercress, tough stems
  trimmed
1 Belgian endive, cut crosswise into 1/2-in.
  (1-cm) wide strips
1 head Bibb lettuce, separated into leaves

1. With small paring knife, peel grapefruits. Working over bowl to catch juice, separate grapefruit sections from membranes; reserve juice that collects in bowl.

2. In medium bowl, whisk together mayonnaise, chutney, mustard, sesame oil, salt, pepper and 3 tbsp (45 mL) of reserved grapefruit juice.

3. Add crabmeat, tossing to combine. Add watercress, endive and grapefruit sections, and toss. Serve salad on bed of Bibb lettuce.

Calories: 180, fat: 4 g, saturated fat: 1 g, sodium: 660 mg, carbohydrate: 20 g, protein: 18 g.

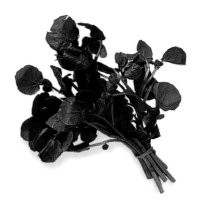

Cold Tuna & Vegetable Salad

This salad offers omega-3 fatty acids from the tuna and lots of vitamins C and B₆.

PREPARATION TIME: 45 MINUTES • SERVES 4

1 lb (500 g) small red or white new potatoes
2 oz (60 g, or about 1 cup/250 mL) thin
  green beans
2 large eggs
1/2 lb (250 g) mixed lettuce leaves, washed
1 tbsp (15 mL) chopped parsley
1 tbsp (15 mL) snipped fresh chives
1 small red onion, sliced thin
1 tbsp (15 mL) bottled tapenade
2 garlic cloves, minced
2 tbsp (25 mL) extra-virgin olive oil
1 tbsp (15 mL) red wine vinegar
1 tsp (5 mL) balsamic vinegar
10 or 15 radishes, sliced thin
1 can (6 oz/175 g) tuna packed in water,
  drained
1/2 cup (125 mL) cherry tomatoes
1 red bell pepper, seeded and sliced thin
1 yellow pepper, seeded and sliced thin
1 green pepper, seeded and sliced thin
8 black olives
Fresh basil leaves, for garnish

1. Put potatoes in pot with water to cover and bring to boil. Simmer 10 minutes, add beans and cook until vegetables are tender, 5 minutes. Drain and rinse under cold water.

2. Put eggs in small pot with cold water to cover; bring to boil. Simmer gently for 5 minutes, drain, and rinse under cold water. Peel eggs and let stand in a bowl of cold water.

3. In large, shallow bowl, toss together lettuce, parsley, chives and red onion.

4. In small bowl, whisk together tapenade, garlic, olive oil, vinegars, salt and pepper to taste. Pour two-thirds of dressing over salad and toss.

5. Halve potatoes and arrange on top of salad with green beans, radishes, chunks of tuna, tomatoes, peppers and olives. Quarter eggs and add to the salad. Pour remaining dressing on top and garnish with basil leaves.

Calories: 350, fat: 15 g, saturated fat: 3 g, sodium: 450 mg, carbohydrate: 36 g, protein: 18 g.

Spinach Salad with Chickpeas

Forget the heavy spinach salads loaded with fat and cholesterol. Fresh and delicious, this crunchy salad is packed with antioxidants, fibre, and cancer-fighting ingredients.

PREPARATION TIME: 10 MINUTES

COOKING TIME: 20 MINUTES • SERVES 4

2 medium onions, cut into
    ½-inch (1-cm) slices
1 can (19 oz/540 mL) chickpeas, drained,
    rinsed, and patted dry
¼ cup (50 mL) lemon juice
2 tbsp (25 mL) flaxseed oil
1 tbsp (15 mL) olive oil
1 clove garlic, minced
½ tsp (2 mL) salt
¼ cup (50 mL) crumbled feta cheese
1 package (7 oz/198 g) baby spinach
2 apples, cored and sliced
2 tbsp (25 mL) ground flaxseed

1. Preheat oven to 400°F (200°C). Coat baking sheet with olive oil cooking spray. Add onion slices and coat each with spray. Roast 10 minutes. Add chickpeas and roast until onions are tender and browned, 10 minutes.

2. Meanwhile, in measuring cup, whisk together lemon juice, flaxseed oil, olive oil, garlic and salt. Stir in cheese.

3. Place spinach in large bowl and toss with onions, chickpeas, apples and flaxseed. Drizzle with vinaigrette.

Calories: 292, fat: 14 g, saturated fat: 3 g, sodium: 476 mg, carbohydrate: 37 g, protein: 18 g.

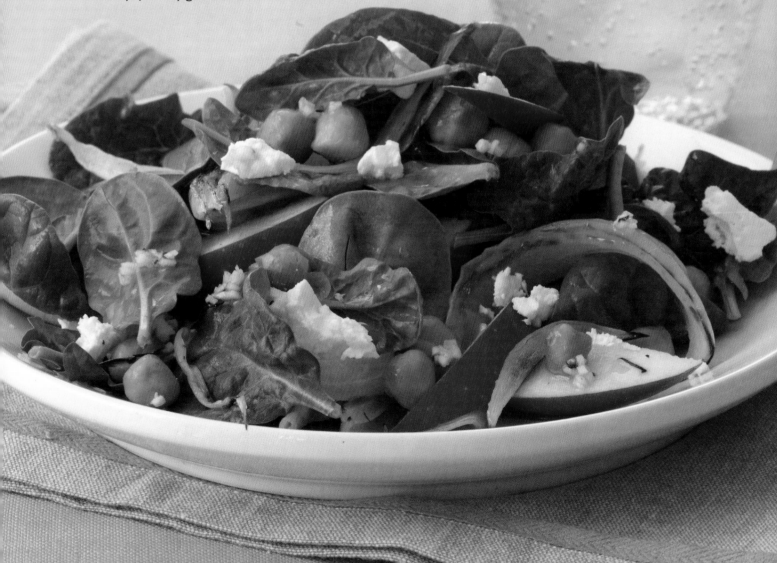

Smoked Turkey & Melon Salad

Powerful portions of vitamins E and C star in this cool main-dish salad that takes the edge off hot weather.

PREPARATION TIME: 20 MINUTES • SERVES 4

3 cups (750 mL) honeydew and/or cantaloupe balls

³/₄ lb (375 g) smoked turkey breast, cut into ¹/₂-in. (1-cm) cubes

¹/₂ cup (125 mL) thinly sliced celery

2 scallions, sliced

2 tbsp (25 mL) slivered fresh basil

2 tbsp (25 mL) chopped toasted walnuts or pecans

2 tbsp (25 mL) honey mustard

1 tbsp (15 mL) white wine vinegar

2 tsp (10 mL) olive oil

¹/₂ tsp (2 mL) soy sauce

1. In large bowl, toss together melon balls, turkey, celery, scallions, basil and walnuts.

2. In small bowl, whisk together honey mustard, vinegar, oil and soy sauce. Toss dressing with melon mixture just before serving.

Calories: 210, fat: 8 g, saturated fat: 2 g, sodium: 850 mg, carbohydrate: 23 g, protein: 16 g.

Warm Snow Pea Salad with Mushrooms & Goat Cheese

Snow peas and watercress offer calcium and vitamin C, while mushrooms supply vitamin D. Red peppers give you more vitamin C and the goat cheese ups your total of calcium for this delectable salad. Pecans supply omega-3 fatty acids.

PREPARATION TIME: 15 MINUTES

COOKING TIME: 10 MINUTES • SERVES 4

2 tsp (10 mL) olive oil

¹/₂ lb (250 g) mushrooms, thinly sliced

2 cloves garlic, minced

1 lb (500 g) snow peas, strings removed

1 small red bell pepper, cut into 2-in. x ¹/₄-in (5-cm x 0.5-cm) strips

¹/₂ tsp (2 mL) salt

3 tbsp (45 mL) rice vinegar

2 tsp (10 mL) honey

4 cups (1 L) watercress leaves

4 oz (125 g) mild goat cheese

2 tbsp (25 mL) pecans, toasted and chopped

1. In large nonstick skillet, over moderately high heat, heat 1 tsp (15 mL) of oil. Add mushrooms and sauté for 4 minutes or until tender and lightly browned. Add garlic and cook 1 minute. Add snow peas, bell pepper and salt, and sauté for 4 minutes or until crisp-tender.

2. Transfer to a large bowl and add vinegar, honey and remaining 1 tsp (15 mL) oil, tossing to combine. Let stand for 20 minutes before serving.

3. Divide watercress among 4 salad plates and top with snow pea mixture. Sprinkle with goat cheese and pecans.

Calories: 240, fat: 14 g, saturated fat: 6 g, sodium: 400 mg, carbohydrate: 19 g, protein: 12 g.

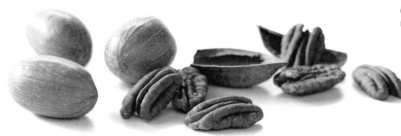

Grilled Steak & Vegetables

The vegetables offer up the main nutritional benefits—vitamin C, folate and vitamin B₆—in this delightful barbecue. The canola oil adds omega-3 fatty acids, the beef adds more vitamin B₆, and the dish fits in with a low-calorie diet.

PREPARATION TIME: 20 MINUTES PLUS MARINATING TIME • COOKING TIME: 20 MINUTES • SERVES 4

4 lean London broil steaks (4 oz/125 g each)
3 tbsp (45 mL) canola oil
3 tbsp (45 mL) red wine vinegar
2 tbsp (25 mL) Dijon mustard
2 cloves garlic, finely chopped
1 tsp (5 mL) each dried basil and oregano
1/8 tsp (0.5 mL) hot red pepper flakes
1/8 tsp (0.5 mL) each salt and freshly ground black pepper
2 red or green bell peppers, cut lengthwise into 1-in. (2.5-cm) strips
3 zucchini, each cut lengthwise into 4 strips
2 red or yellow onions, cut across into 1/2-in. (1-cm) slices

1. Using a sharp knife, trim fat from steaks.

2. For marinade: In small bowl, mix oil with vinegar, mustard, garlic, basil, oregano, hot pepper flakes, salt and pepper.

3. Place steaks in dish just large enough to hold them and pour two-thirds of marinade over. Turn meat in marinade to coat. Cover dish and marinate in refrigerator at least 2 hours.

4. Remove meat from refrigerator and allow to come to room temperature. Pour off marinade and discard. Preheat a charcoal grill or broiler, setting rack 4 to 5 in. (10 to 12 cm) from the heat.

5. Add steaks to grill or broiler and cook according to taste, about 6 minutes per side for medium. Meanwhile, using a small brush, coat vegetable pieces with remaining marinade mixture.

6. Transfer steaks to platter, cover with foil, and keep warm. Add vegetables to grill or broiler and cook until browned and softened, turning once and brushing twice with remaining marinade.

Calories: 327, fat: 18 g, saturated fat: 6 g, sodium: 271 mg, carbohydrate: 16 g, protein: 27 g.

Italian Beef & Broccoli Sauté

Broccoli, tomatoes, and peppers give this low-calorie dinner high marks for vitamin C. Broccoli adds plenty of calcium and the beef some vitamin B₆.

PREPARATION TIME: 25 MINUTES

COOKING TIME: 20 MINUTES • SERVES 4

3 pickled red cherry peppers
3/4 lb (375 g) well-trimmed beef sirloin, thinly sliced
2 tbsp (25 mL) balsamic vinegar
2 cloves garlic, minced
2 tsp (10 mL) olive oil
1 red onion, thinly sliced
1 yellow or red bell pepper, slivered
6 cups (1.5 L) small broccoli florets
3/4 tsp (4 mL) dried oregano
2 cups (500 mL) cherry tomatoes, halved
1/3 cup (75 mL) chopped fresh basil
1/2 tsp (2 mL) salt

1. Mince one cherry pepper. In medium bowl, combine minced pepper, beef, vinegar and garlic. Let stand 15 minutes. Meanwhile, dice remaining cherry peppers.

2. In large skillet, heat oil over moderate heat. Add onion and bell pepper, and cook 5 minutes. Add broccoli and oregano, reduce heat to moderately low, cover, and cook, stirring occasionally, 10 minutes or until broccoli is crisp-tender.

3. Push vegetables to one side, increase heat to moderately high, and add reserved cherry peppers and beef with marinade. Sauté for 2 minutes. Add cherry tomatoes, basil and salt, and sauté for 2 minutes or until heated through.

Calories: 280, fat: 12 g, saturated fat: 4 g, sodium: 330 mg, carbohydrate: 17 g, protein: 29 g.

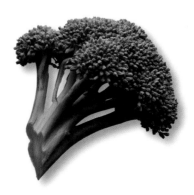

recipes for beating arthritis   **227**

Spicy Lamb Stew with Couscous

Capture the atmosphere of Morocco with this vitamin-filled stew, called a tagine, in which zucchini, carrots, tomatoes, onions, and apricots all contribute vitamin C and several contribute folate and/or vitamin E.

PREPARATION TIME: 35 MINUTES

COOKING TIME: 2 HOURS • SERVES 6

1³⁄₄ lb (795 g) boneless leg of lamb, trimmed and cut into 1-in. (2.5-cm) cubes
1 small onion, chopped
2 cloves garlic, chopped
¹⁄₂ tsp (2 mL) cayenne pepper
1 cinnamon stick, broken in half
1 tsp (5 mL) ground ginger
1 tsp (5 mL) sweet paprika
¹⁄₄ tsp (1 mL) crumbled saffron threads
³⁄₄ cup (175 mL) dried apricots, quartered
1 cup (250 mL) chopped carrots
1 cup (250 mL) chopped zucchini
2 medium tomatoes, chopped
3 tbsp (45 mL) chopped fresh coriander
3 tbsp (45 mL) chopped fresh parsley
1¹⁄₂ cups (375 mL) (about 10 oz/300 g) couscous

1. In a large pot, combine lamb, onion, garlic, cayenne pepper, cinnamon, ginger, paprika, saffron, and salt and pepper to taste. Add enough water to cover and simmer mixture, covered, for 1 hour 30 minutes.

2. Add apricots, carrots, zucchini, tomatoes, 2 tbsp (25 mL) coriander and 2 tbsp (25 mL) parsley to pan and simmer, covered, 15 minutes more.

3. Meanwhile, put couscous in a bowl, add just enough cold water to cover it and let it stand for 5 minutes to absorb the liquid.

4. Transfer couscous to a sieve, and steam couscous over stew until warm, about 15 minutes. Fluff with fork and add salt to taste.

5. To serve, spoon couscous onto serving dish. Using a slotted spoon, top couscous with lamb and vegetables and sprinkle with remaining coriander and parsley. Serve cooking liquid on side as a sauce.

Calories: 420, fat: 7 g, saturated fat: 2 g, sodium: 100 mg, carbohydrate: 54 g, protein: 35 g.

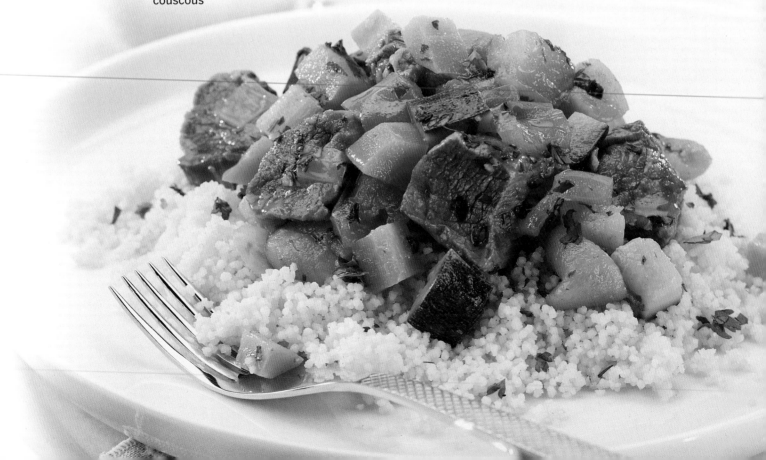

Lamb Curry

In this mild curry, lean lamb gives you vitamin B₆ and folate; the yogourt gives calcium; the onions and tomato paste give vitamins C, E, and folate.

PREPARATION TIME: 15 MINUTES

COOKING TIME: 1 HOUR 10 MINUTES • SERVES 4

⅓ cup (75 mL) plain low-fat yogourt
½ tsp (2 mL) cayenne pepper
2 tsp (10 mL) ground coriander
1½ tsp (7 mL) ground cumin
2 tsp (10 mL) crushed garlic
2 tsp (10 mL) grated fresh ginger
1 tsp (5 mL) sweet paprika
½ tsp (2 mL) ground turmeric
1¼ lb (625 g) boneless leg of lamb, trimmed and cut into 2-in. (5-cm) cubes
1¾ cups (425 mL) finely chopped onion
1½ tbsp (20 mL) tomato paste
Salt to taste
2 tbsp (25 mL) unsalted butter
2 bay leaves
2 green cardamom pods, tops split open
1 cinnamon stick, broken in half
4 whole cloves
½ tsp (2 mL) freshly grated nutmeg
1 tbsp (15 mL) chopped fresh mint
2 tbsp (25 mL) chopped fresh coriander

1. In small bowl, combine first 8 ingredients.

2. In nonstick pot, medium heat, cook lamb and onions, stirring until meat begins to sizzle.

3. Add yogourt mixture. Over low heat, cook, covered, stirring occasionally, until lamb releases its juices, about 30 minutes. Cook uncovered, medium heat, stirring, until sauce reduces to pastelike consistency, 5–6 minutes.

4. Stir in tomato paste, salt and 1 tbsp (15 mL) butter. Reduce heat to low and cook, uncovered, 3 minutes. Stir in ¾ cup (175 mL) boiling water and simmer, covered, 15 minutes.

5. In small skillet, low heat, melt 1 tbsp (15 mL) butter. Add bay leaves, cardamom, cinnamon and cloves and sizzle for 30 seconds. Add nutmeg, stir once; pour over meat. Stir well and simmer, covered, 10 minutes. Stir in mint and coriander.

Calories: 300, fat: 13 g, saturated fat: 6 g, sodium: 135 mg, carbohydrate: 12 g, protein: 32 g.

Mediterranean Lamb Roast & Potatoes

This one-dish meal is an easy Greek-style roast bursting with the fresh flavours of lemon and herbs and offering an array of arthritis-healthy nutrients. You will get vitamin B₆ and folate from the lamb, vitamins C and E from the tomatoes, vitamin C and folate from the onions or shallots, vitamins B₆ and C from the potatoes, and vitamin C from the lemon.

PREPARATION TIME: 15-20 MINUTES

COOKING TIME: 1 HOUR-1 HOUR, 5 MINUTES • SERVES 4

1¼ lb (625 g) boneless leg of lamb, trimmed and cut into 1-in. (2.5-cm) cubes
2 medium onions, cut into quarters
1¼ lb (625 g) small new potatoes, scrubbed and halved if large
1 large lemon, cut into 8 wedges
1 tbsp (15 mL) olive oil
12 garlic cloves, peeled
6 sprigs fresh rosemary
6 sprigs fresh thyme
⅓ lb (150 g) cherry or grape tomatoes, halved
1 tbsp (15 mL) bottled mint sauce, or 2 tbsp (25 mL) mint jelly, melted

1. Preheat oven to 400°F (200°C).

2. Arrange lamb, onions and potatoes in large roasting pan. Squeeze juice from four lemon wedges over meat and vegetables, and drizzle with oil. Tuck lemon wedges, garlic and half of herbs among meat and vegetables and season with salt and pepper. Cover tightly with foil and roast 45 minutes.

3. Remove pan from oven, discard foil and herbs, and increase oven to 425°F (220°C). Add tomatoes, remaining herbs and mint sauce or jelly and toss meat and vegetables well. Roast, uncovered, until meat and vegetables are browned and tender, 15 to 20 minutes.

Calories: 420, fat: 10 g, saturated fat: 3 g, sodium: 105 mg, carbohydrate: 49 g, protein: 34 g.

Spinach-Stuffed Meat Loaf

Spinach is a superfood for people with arthritis— with vitamins B_6, C, E, folate and calcium. Beef and turkey add to the vitamin B_6. Ricotta shores you up with calcium, and the onions, tomatoes and carrots together give you lots of vitamin C and some vitamin E and folate.

PREPARATION TIME: 130 MINUTES

COOKING TIME: 1½ HOURS • SERVES 6

1 lb (500 g) lean ground beef
8 oz (250 g) lean ground turkey
1 small onion, finely chopped
½ cup (125 mL) fresh bread crumbs
⅛ tsp (0.5 mL) garlic salt
1 tbsp (15 mL) tomato paste
1 egg white
½ cup (125 mL) part-skim ricotta cheese
1 package (10 oz/300 g) frozen chopped
    spinach, thawed and drained
⅛ tsp (0.5 mL) each salt and pepper
2 large onions, thinly sliced
2 carrots, coarsely chopped
1 can (28 oz/796 mL) crushed tomatoes

1. In bowl, mix beef, turkey, chopped onion, bread crumbs, garlic salt and tomato paste. In another bowl, mix egg white, ricotta, spinach, salt and pepper.

2. Preheat oven to 350°F (180°C). Turn out beef mixture onto large sheet of wax paper, and form into a 9-in. x 10-in. (23-cm x 25-cm) rectangle.

3. Spoon spinach stuffing lengthwise down centre of meat, leaving about 1 in. (2.5 cm) uncovered at each short end.

4. With help of wax paper, lift long edges of meat. Fold meat over stuffing to enclose it.

5. Pinch edges of meat together. Place loaf seam side down in nonstick roasting pan. Add onions, carrots and tomatoes to pan.

6. Bake about 1½ hours or until meat and vegetables are cooked. Transfer meat to platter. Purée vegetables in a blender and serve sauce with meat loaf.

Calories: 294, fat: 6 g, saturated fat: 2 g, sodium: 405 mg, carbohydrate: 28 g, protein: 32 g.

Beef & Turkey Chili

Both beef and turkey provide you with vitamin B_6; the kidney beans are a prime source of folate; the tomatoes give you vitamins C and E; the onions, peppers, and corn give you more vitamin C and folate. That makes for a hearty and healthy chili!

PREPARATION TIME: 20 MINUTES

COOKING TIME: 50-60 MINUTES • SERVES 6

1 lb (500 g) lean ground beef
8 oz (250 g) lean ground turkey
1 tbsp (15 mL) canola oil
2 large onions, coarsely chopped
3 cloves garlic, finely chopped
3 sweet red or green peppers, coarsely
    chopped
1 tbsp (15 mL) chili powder or to taste
1 tsp (5 mL) each ground cumin and coriander
1 can (28 oz/796 mL) crushed tomatoes
⅛ tsp (0.5 mL) pepper
1 package (10 oz/300 g) frozen corn kernels,
    thawed
1 can (16 oz/453 g) red kidney beans,
    drained and rinsed

1. Heat Dutch oven over moderately high heat. Add beef and turkey and sauté, stirring frequently, about 7 minutes or until meat has lost pink colour and released juices.

2. Remove from heat and spoon meat into sieve set over a bowl. Allow all fat to drain from meat; at least 10 minutes.

3. Meanwhile, in Dutch oven, heat oil over moderate heat. Add onions and garlic and sauté 5 to 7 minutes or until softened and golden brown.

4. Stir in sweet peppers, chili powder and spices, and cook about 5 minutes or until peppers are slightly soft. Return meat to Dutch oven.

5. Stir in crushed tomatoes and pepper, and bring to a boil. Partially cover and simmer, stirring occasionally, 20 to 30 minutes or until sauce thickens.

6. Stir in corn kernels and kidney beans. Cover and cook about 5 minutes to heat through.

Calories: 340, fat: 7 g, saturated fat: 2 g, sodium: 546 mg, carbohydrate: 37 g, protein: 34 g.

Chicken Stew with Balsamic Vinegar

Balsamic vinegar brings a new twist to a classic!

PREPARATION TIME: 15 MINUTES

COOKING TIME: 40 MINUTES • SERVES 4

1 slice thick-cut bacon (2 oz/60 g)

1 broiler-fryer (3 lb/1.5 kg) chicken, skinned and cut into serving-size pieces

1/4 tsp (1 mL) each salt and black pepper

1 package (10 oz/300 g) frozen pearl onions

8 oz (250 g) small mushrooms, quartered

1/4 cup (50 mL) balsamic vinegar

1/2 cup (125 mL) dry red wine

1 1/2 cups (375 mL) chicken stock

1 can (14 oz/398 mL) low-sodium tomatoes, drained and chopped

1 tsp (5 mL) each dried rosemary and thyme, crumbled

1 tbsp (15 mL) cornstarch mixed with 2 tbsp (25 mL) water

2 tbsp (25 mL) minced fresh parsley

1. In nonstick skillet, cook bacon over moderate heat 2 minutes or until crisp. Drain bacon on paper towels, then crumble and set aside. Discard all but 1 tbsp (15 mL) fat. Sprinkle chicken with 1/8 tsp (0.5 mL) each salt and pepper. Set skillet over moderate heat; when bacon fat is hot, sauté chicken until lightly browned, then transfer to 5-qt (5-L) Dutch oven.

2. Add onions, mushrooms and remaining salt and pepper to skillet and sauté, stirring occasionally, for 5 minutes. Transfer vegetables to bowl. Add vinegar and wine to skillet; bring to boil over moderately high heat. Boil mixture, stirring, 1 minute; add to Dutch oven.

3. Add stock, tomatoes, rosemary and thyme to Dutch oven; bring to a boil. Cover, simmer over low heat until meat is no longer pink inside, 15 minutes. Transfer breast pieces to plate; add onions and mushrooms to Dutch oven. Cover, simmer until juices run clear, 8–10 minutes.

4. Return breast pieces to Dutch oven and bring liquid to a boil. Stir in arrowroot mixture and simmer over low heat until the sauce has thickened, 2 to 3 minutes. Sprinkle with tarragon.

Calories: 380, fat: 13 g, saturated fat: 4 g, sodium: 578 mg, carbohydrate: 16 g, protein: 45 g.

Grilled Chicken with Herbs

A tasty chicken that gives you vitamin B_6 is marinated in canola oil, with its omega-3 fatty acids, and herbs to give the chicken a lovely flavour.

PREPARATION TIME: 15 MINUTES • COOKING TIME:

30 MINUTES • MARINRATE 4 HOURS • SERVES 4

1 chicken (about 3 1/2 lb/1.5 kg), cut into serving pieces, wings reserved for another use

3 cloves garlic, finely chopped

3 tbsp (45 mL) chopped parsley

2 tbsp (25 mL) chopped basil

2 tbsp (25 mL) chopped mint

1/3 cup (75 mL) canola oil

1/2 tsp (2 mL) pepper

1/8 tsp (0.5 mL) salt

1. Loosen skin of chicken with tip of a sharp knife, then pull off. Cut off fat and make 2 to 3 slashes in each piece .

2. For marinade: In small bowl, combine garlic with parsley, basil, mint, oil, pepper and salt.

3. Place chicken in large dish, add marinade, and coat chicken. Cover and marinate in refrigerator 4 hours, turning occasionally.

4. Prepare grill or preheat broiler, setting rack 4 in. (10 cm) from heat. Arrange chicken pieces bone side down on grill or broiler rack, reserving marinade. Grill chicken 20 minutes or until browned on one side, brushing once with reserved marinade. Turn pieces over, brush with remaining marinade, and grill 10 minutes longer or until cooked through and juices run clear.

Calories: 306, fat: 15 g, saturated fat: 3 g, sodium: 208 mg, carbohydrate: 2g, protein: 40 g.

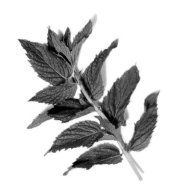

Spicy Asian Chicken Braised with Mushrooms

Hoisin sauce is made from soybeans, garlic, chilis, and other seasonings. It's a potent source of vitamin E and calcium. Mushrooms will give you vitamin D, which helps your body absorb calcium. Rounding out the benefits of this dish are the chicken pieces that give you vitamin B₆ and the peppers that give you B₆, C, and folate.

PREPARATION TIME: 15 MINUTES

COOKING TIME: 40 MINUTES • SERVES 4

3 scallions, thinly sliced
3 cloves garlic, crushed and peeled
3 slices (¼-in/0.5-cm thick) fresh ginger
¼ cup (50 mL) lower-sodium soy sauce
¼ cup (50 mL) hoisin sauce
¼ cup (50 mL) chicken broth
1 tbsp (15 mL) sesame oil
1 tsp (5 mL) crushed red pepper flakes
1 tsp (5 mL) sugar
¾ tsp (4 mL) salt
8 chicken drumsticks (about 2½ lb/1.25 kg), skin removed
1 lb (500 g) mushrooms, quartered
1 large green bell pepper, cut into ½-in. (1-cm) pieces
1½ tsp (7 mL) cornstarch blended with 1 tbsp (15 mL) water
1 cup (250 mL) rice

1. In Dutch oven, stir together scallions, garlic, ginger, soy sauce, hoisin sauce, broth, sesame oil, red pepper flakes, sugar and ¼ tsp (1 mL) salt. Stir in chicken, mushrooms and bell pepper.

2. Bring to boil over medium heat. Reduce heat and simmer, covered, 35 minutes or until chicken is cooked through and vegetables are tender. Stir in cornstarch mixture and cook, stirring constantly, 1 minute or until slightly thickened.

3. Meanwhile, in medium covered pot, bring 2 ¼ cups (550 mL) water to a boil. Add rice and remaining ½ tsp (2 mL) salt. Reduce heat to a simmer, cover, and cook 17 minutes or until rice is tender. Serve sauce and chicken with rice.

Calories: 490, fat: 10 g, saturated fat: 2 g, sodium: 1561 mg, carbohydrate: 58 g, protein: 39 g.

Pesto Chicken on Focaccia

In Italy, a slice of focaccia is a popular snack. When you add vitamin B₆-rich chicken to this thick slice of bread, along with calcium-rich cheese, vitamin E-rich nuts, and peppers with their vitamins B₆ and C, as well as folate, you are talking serious good nutrition for someone with arthritis.

PREPARATION TIME: 15 MINUTES

COOKING TIME: 15 MINUTES • SERVES 4

1 clove garlic, peeled
½ cup (125 mL) packed fresh basil leaves
3 tbsp (45 mL) grated Parmesan cheese
1 tbsp (15 mL) plus 2 tsp (10 mL) olive oil
2 tbsp (25 mL) slivered almonds
¼ tsp (1 mL) salt
1 round focaccia (10-in./25-cm diameter, 8 oz/250 g)
2 cups (500 mL) mixed greens
2 cooked skinless, boneless chicken breast halves (leftover or poached), thinly sliced crosswise on the diagonal
½ cup (125 mL) bottled roasted red peppers, cut into thin strips

1. Preheat oven to 400°F (200°C). To make pesto: In small pan of boiling water, blanch garlic 1 minute. Drain and transfer to food processor. Add basil, Parmesan, oil, almonds, salt and 2 tbsp (25 mL) of water, and process until smooth.

2. Bake focaccia for 10 minutes. When cool enough to handle, slice in half horizontally. Spread pesto onto both focaccia halves. Top with mixed greens. Place chicken and roasted peppers on top of greens. Cover with focaccia top. To serve, cut into 4 wedges.

Calories: 356, fat: 13 g, saturated fat: 3 g, sodium: 599 mg, carbohydrate: 30 g, protein: 30 g.

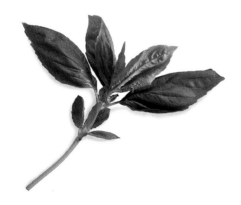

Poached Chicken

This simple recipe covers quite a few nutritional bases: The chicken gives you vitamin B_6; the carrots give you vitamin C; the potatoes give you a little more of each. Plus, the leeks and lemon juice add to the vitamin C count.

PREPARATION TIME: 25-30 MINUTES • COOKING TIME:

$1\frac{1}{4}$-$1\frac{1}{2}$ HOURS MOSTLY UNATTENDED • SERVES 4

1 whole chicken ($3\frac{1}{2}$ pounds/1.75 kg)
6 cups (1.5 L) chicken stock
5 cups (1.25 L) water
4 carrots, cut into 1-in. (2.5-cm) pieces
2 leeks, white part only, sliced
2 large potatoes, peeled and cut into cubes
6 cloves garlic, peeled
1 bouquet garni, made with 8 sprigs parsley and 2 bay leaves
1 tbsp (15 mL) lemon juice
$\frac{1}{8}$ tsp (0.5 mL) each salt and pepper

1. Cut fat from both ends of bird and wipe inside with paper towel. Tuck wings under bird. Fold skin over body cavity opening; tie legs together with string.

2. Place chicken in a 4-qt (4-L) Dutch oven. Add stock and water to cover. Bring to a boil over moderate heat and, using a large spoon, skim off scum.

3. Add vegetables, garlic and herbs to Dutch oven and simmer, partially covered, $1\frac{1}{4}$ hours or until chicken and vegetables are cooked through.

4. Transfer chicken to platter, cover with aluminum foil, and keep warm. Strain stock into a bowl and skim off fat. Reserve vegetables and discard herbs.

5. In a blender or food processor, purée half of vegetables and $1\frac{1}{2}$ cups (375 mL) stock; pour into pan. Add lemon juice, salt and pepper.

6. Remove skin from chicken and carve meat. Meanwhile, warm sauce gently. Place chicken and remaining vegetables on platter and pour sauce over.

Calories: 299, fat: 7 g, saturated fat: 2 g, sodium: 354 mg, carbohydrate: 30 g, protein: 47 g.

Sesame Chicken Salad

The perfect summer entrée, this Chinese-style chicken and vegetable salad offers plenty of calcium from snow peas, vitamin C from peppers and snow peas, and vitamin B_6 from snow peas and chicken.

PREPARATION TIME: 20 MINUTES

COOKING TIME: 2 MINUTES • SERVES 4

2 cloves garlic, peeled
$\frac{1}{2}$ lb (250 g) snow peas, strings removed
1 red bell pepper, cut into 2-in. (5-cm)-long matchsticks
1 piece (2 in./5 cm) fresh ginger, peeled and thickly sliced
3 tbsp (45 mL) sesame oil
3 tbsp (45 mL) lower-sodium soy sauce
$2\frac{1}{2}$ tsp (12 mL) sugar
$2\frac{1}{2}$ tsp (12 mL) rice vinegar
$\frac{1}{4}$ tsp (1 mL) crushed red pepper flakes
1 cucumber, peeled, halved lengthwise, seeded and cut into 2-in. (5-cm) long matchsticks
2 cups (500 mL) shredded cooked chicken breasts or thighs—leftover or poached

1. In large pot of boiling water, blanch garlic 1 minute; remove with slotted spoon. Add snow peas and bell pepper, and blanch 15 seconds; drain well.

2. In food processor, combine blanched garlic, ginger, sesame oil, soy sauce, sugar, vinegar and red pepper flakes, and process until smooth.

3. Transfer dressing to large bowl. Add snow peas, bell pepper, cucumber and chicken, and toss to combine. Serve at room temperature or chilled.

Calories: 263, fat: 13 g, saturated fat: 2 g, sodium: 508 mg, carbohydrate: 12 g, protein: 25 g.

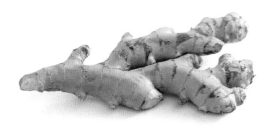

Thai Chicken Stew

Thai cooking demands a careful balance of tastes and textures. There is also a balance of nutrients: vitamin E and calcium from the soy milk; vitamin B₆ from the chicken, bell pepper, potatoes, and peanut butter; vitamin C from the bell pepper, potatoes, and lime juice, and folate from the peanut butter.

PREPARATION TIME: 25 MINUTES

COOKING TIME: 20 MINUTES • SERVES 4

2 tsp (10 mL) vegetable oil

1 red bell pepper, cut into ½-in. (1-cm) squares

2 cloves garlic, minced

1 tbsp (15 mL) minced fresh ginger

¾ lb (375 g) all-purpose potatoes (2 to 3 medium), peeled and cut into ½-in. (1-cm) chunks

1 cup (250 mL) chicken broth

1 lb (500 g) skinless, boneless chicken breasts, cut into 1-in. (2.5-cm) chunks

2 cups (500 mL) unflavoured soy milk

⅓ cup (75 mL) chopped fresh basil

¼ cup (50 mL) chopped cilantro

2 tbsp (25 mL) lime juice

2 tbsp (25 mL) lower-sodium soy sauce

1 tbsp (15 mL) reduced-fat peanut butter

2 tsp (10 mL) dark brown sugar

¼ tsp (1 mL) coconut extract

1. In large nonstick skillet, heat oil over moderate heat. Add bell pepper, garlic and ginger, and sauté for 4 minutes or until pepper is crisp-tender. Add potatoes and broth, and bring to a boil. Reduce to a simmer, cover, and cook 7 minutes or until potatoes are firm-tender.

2. Add chicken, soy milk, basil, cilantro, lime juice, soy sauce, peanut butter, brown sugar and coconut extract to pan, and bring to a boil. Reduce to a simmer, cover, and cook 5 minutes or until chicken and potatoes are cooked through.

Calories: 430, fat: 21 g, saturated fat: 6 g, sodium: 410 mg, carbohydrate: 34 g, protein: 27 g.

Jamaican Jerked Chicken Salad

Assemble this salad at serving time, because an enzyme in kiwis, actinidin, quickly starts to break down any protein it happens to be in contact with. If the chicken and kiwi sit too long, the chicken begins to get mushy, so eat this spicy and refreshing salad while the chicken is still warm.

PREPARATION TIME: 10 MINUTES

COOKING TIME: 8 MINUTES • SERVES 4

4 scallions, thinly sliced

3 cloves garlic, minced

¼ tsp (1 mL) dried thyme

1 tsp (5 mL) black pepper

I tsp (5 mL) ground allspice

I tsp (5 mL) salt

4 tbsp (60 mL) red wine vinegar

2 tbsp (35 mL) Dijon mustard

2 tsp (10 mL) dark brown sugar

1 lb (500 g) skinless, boneless chicken breasts

1 tbsp (15 mL) olive oil

2 cups (500 mL) pineapple chunks

4 kiwis, peeled and cut into wedges

1 large red bell pepper, cut into matchsticks

1 cup (250 mL) jicama matchsticks

1. In a large bowl, stir together garlic, thyme, black pepper, allspice, half the scallions and ½ tsp (2 mL) salt. Stir in 2 tbsp (25 mL) of the vinegar, 1 tbsp (15 mL) mustard, and brown sugar. Add chicken, rubbing mixture into meat. Cover and set aside.

2. In separate bowl, whisk together remaining vinegar, mustard, ¼ tsp (1 mL) salt and oil. Add remaining scallions, pineapple, kiwis, bell pepper and jicama, and toss.

3. Preheat broiler. Broil chicken 6 in. (15 cm) from heat, 4 minutes per side, or until cooked through. When cool enough to handle, slice chicken on the diagonal. Add to bowl and toss.

Calories: 287, fat: 5.6 g, saturated fat: 0.8 g, sodium: 213 mg, carbohydrate: 31 g, protein: 28 g.

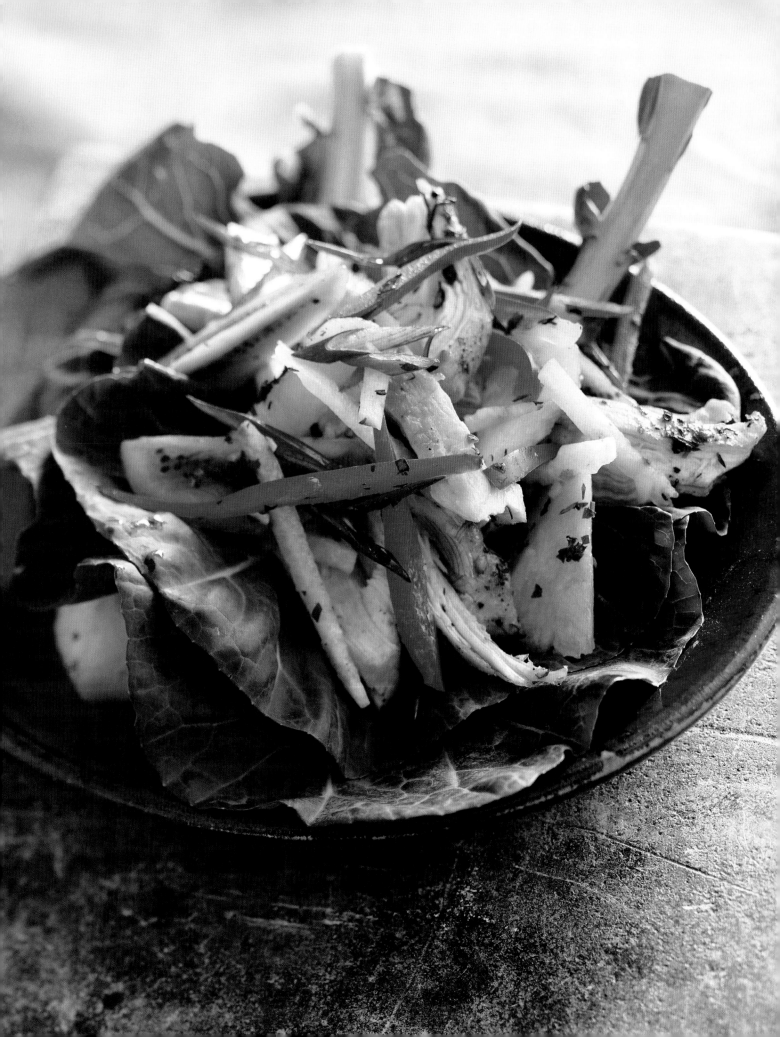

Turkey Quesadillas

This spicy Southwestern dish can also be made with ground chicken, beef or pork, which give you vitamin B₆ just like the turkey. The peppers and onions offer vitamin C and folate, and the cheese provides calcium.

PREPARATION TIME: 20 MINUTES

COOKING TIME: 25 MINUTES • SERVES 6

6 flour tortillas, 7 in. (18 cm) in diameter
2 tsp (10 mL) olive oil
1 medium yellow onion, finely chopped (1 cup)
1 medium sweet red pepper, cored, seeded and diced ($3/4$ cup/175 mL)
1¼ lb (625 g) ground turkey
¼ tsp (1 mL) salt
2 cloves garlic, minced
1 tsp (5 mL) each ground cumin, chili powder and dried oregano, crumbled
1 jalapeño pepper, seeded and finely chopped (1 tbsp/15 mL)
½ cup (125 mL) low-sodium tomato sauce
2 tbsp (25 mL) minced fresh cilantro (coriander) or 2 tbsp (25 mL) minced parsley mixed with ¾ tsp (4 mL) dried cilantro
½ cup (125 mL) grated Monterey Jack cheese (2 oz/60 g)
1 cup (250 mL) tomato salsa

1. Preheat oven to 350°F (180°C). Wrap tortillas in aluminum foil and heat in oven 8 minutes. Meanwhile, in 12-in. (30-cm) nonstick skillet, heat oil over moderate heat. Add onion and red pepper and sauté, stirring occasionally, 5 minutes or until onion is soft.

2. Add turkey and salt to skillet and sauté, stirring, 3 minutes or until turkey is no longer pink. Add garlic, cumin, chili powder, oregano and jalapeño pepper; sauté, stirring, 1 minute or until mixture is dry. Stir in tomato sauce and cilantro.

3. Increase oven temperature to 450°F (230°C). Unwrap tortillas and place on greased baking sheets. Spread equal amount of turkey mixture on each and sprinkle with cheese. Bake 8 to 10 minutes or until cheese is melted and tortillas are golden. Serve with salsa.

Calories: 277, fat: 9 g, saturated fat: 1 g, sodium: 213 mg, carbohydrate: 22 g, protein: 26 g.

Salmon Steaks Mexican-Style

A healthy and delicious supplier of omega-3 fatty acids, salmon gets a spicy treatment in this recipe, which also offers lots of vitamin C (tomatoes, onions, lime juice, hot pepper), a little vitamin E (tomatoes), and folate (onions and pepper).

PREPARATION TIME: 15 MINUTES

COOKING TIME: 55 MINUTES • SERVES 4

2 tsp (10 mL) olive oil
1 small onion, finely chopped
2 cloves garlic, minced
1 tsp (5 mL) chili powder
1 can (14 oz/398 mL) no-salt-added tomatoes, chopped, with their juice
1 pickled jalapeño, finely chopped
¼ cup (50 mL) pitted green olives, coarsely chopped
1½ tsp (7 mL) capers, rinsed and drained
¼ tsp (1 mL) each dried oregano and thyme
⅛ tsp (0.5 mL) each cinnamon and salt
4 salmon steaks (8 oz/250 g each)
2 tbsp (25 mL) lime juice

1. In a large nonstick skillet, heat oil over moderate heat. Sauté onion and garlic until soft, 5 minutes. Add chili powder, stirring to coat onions. Add tomatoes, jalapeño, olives, capers, oregano, thyme, cinnamon, salt and ¼ cup (50 mL) water; bring to a boil. Reduce heat, cover, and simmer until sauce is richly flavoured, 30 minutes.

2. Preheat oven to 350°F (180°C). Sprinkle salmon with lime juice; place in a 9-in. × 13-in. (23-cm × 33-cm) baking dish. Spoon ¾ cup (175 mL) sauce over fish and bake until it flakes when tested with a fork, 15–20 minutes. Reheat remaining sauce; spoon over fish.

Calories: 500, fat: 29 g, saturated fat: 5 g, sodium: 530 mg, carbohydrate: 12 g, protein: 46 g.

Broiled Herb-Rubbed Salmon

This simple and speedy way of cooking salmon brings out all its good flavour and gives you a full shot of omega-3 fatty acids.

PREPARATION TIME: 10 MINUTES

COOKING TIME: 5 MINUTES • SERVES 4

3/4 tsp (4 mL) salt
1/2 tsp (2 mL) sugar
1/2 tsp (2 mL) crumbled dried rosemary
1/4 tsp (1 mL) dried tarragon
1 pinch (0.5 mL) ground allspice
4 six-ounce (175-g) salmon fillets

1. Preheat broiler. In small bowl, combine salt, sugar, rosemary, tarragon and ground allspice.

2. Rub mixture into salmon fillets.

3. Broil, skin side down, 6 inches (15 cm) from heat, without turning, 5 minutes or until salmon just flakes when tested with a fork.

Calories: 310, fat: 18 g, saturated fat: 4 g, sodium: 450 mg, carbohydrate: 1 g, protein: 34 g.

Summer Salmon & Asparagus

Fresh young vegetables and succulent salmon make this casserole highly nutritious—in addition to the omega-3 fatty acids supplied by the fish, you gain vitamin C and folate from the leeks, and vitamins C and B$_6$ and folate from the asparagus.

PREPARATION TIME: 10 MINUTES

COOKING TIME: ABOUT 20 MINUTES • SERVES 4

4 skinless salmon fillets (5 oz/150 g each)
7 oz (198 g) baby leeks
8 oz (250 g) tender asparagus spears
5 oz (150 g) sugar snap peas
4 tbsp (60 mL) dry white wine
3/4 cup (175 mL) fish or vegetable stock, preferably fresh stock
2 tbsp (25 mL) butter, diced
Salt and fresh-ground black pepper
1 tbsp (15 mL) snipped fresh chives

1. Run your fingertips over each salmon fillet to check for stray bones, pulling out any that you find. In bottom of large, shallow flameproof casserole, arrange leeks in single layer. Lay salmon fillets on top. Surround fish with asparagus and sugar snap peas. Pour in wine and stock, and dot fish with butter. Season with salt and pepper to taste.

2. Bring to boil, then cover casserole with tight-fitting lid and reduce heat so liquid simmers gently. Simmer fish and vegetables until salmon is pale pink all the way through and vegetables are fork-tender, 12 to 14 minutes. Sprinkle chives over salmon.

Calories: 370, fat: 21 g, saturated fat: 7 g, sodium: 220 mg, carbohydrate: 9 g, protein: 33 g.

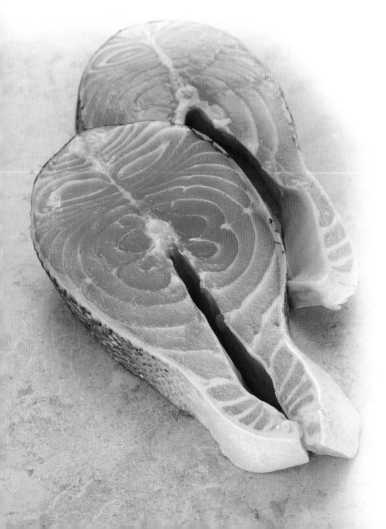

Walnut-Crusted Snapper

Walnuts have vitamin E; snapper fillets, omega-3 fatty acids; lemon juice and zest, vitamin C; and Parmesan, plenty of calcium. This is a terrific low-calorie dinner entrée for watching your weight and your arthritis.

PREPARATION TIME: 15 MINUTES

COOKING TIME: 15 MINUTES • SERVES 4

3 tbsp (45 mL) light mayonnaise
½ tsp (2 mL) grated lemon zest
1 tsp (5 mL) lemon juice
¼ tsp (1 mL) each salt and pepper
4 red snapper fillets (6 oz/175 g each), skinned
½ cup (125 mL) walnut halves
2 tbsp (25 mL) grated Parmesan cheese

1. Preheat oven to 450°F (230°C). Spray large baking sheet with nonstick cooking spray; set aside.

2. In small bowl, combine mayonnaise, lemon zest, lemon juice, salt and pepper. Place fillets, skinned side down, on prepared baking sheet. Spread mayonnaise mixture over fish.

3. In food processor, process walnuts and Parmesan until finely ground (but not pasty). Sprinkle nut mixture over fish, patting it on. Bake for 15 minutes or until nuts are lightly browned and fish is just cooked through or just flakes when tested with a fork.

Calories: 320, fat: 16 g, saturated fat: 2 g, sodium: 370 mg, carbohydrate: 3 g, protein: 40 g.

Garlic, Tomato & Anchovy Toasts

Anchovies give these toasts a sharp, salty taste along with omega-3 fatty acids. The tomatoes and lemon juice add a healthy shot of vitamin C.

PREPARATION TIME: 5 MINUTES PLUS 10 MINUTES

SOAKING • COOKING TIME: 2-3 MINUTES • SERVES 4

3 anchovy fillets
2 tbsp (25 mL) skim milk
1 clove garlic, crushed
1 tsp (5 mL) fresh lemon juice
4 diagonal slices of Italian or French bread, 1 in. (2.5 cm) thick
2 tomatoes, sliced thin
1 tbsp (15 mL) olive oil
Freshly ground black pepper
¼ cup (50 mL) small basil leaves

1. In small dish, soak anchovies in milk for 10 minutes. Drain, rinse and pat fish dry. Mash anchovies, garlic and lemon juice with mortar and pestle or a fork until they form a paste.

2. Preheat broiler with rack set 6 inches (15 cm) from heat. Toast bread on both sides under broiler. Spread one fourth of paste thinly on one side of each slice.

3. Arrange tomato slices on top of toasts. Drizzle with oil, season with pepper and place on baking sheet. Broil until tomatoes are softened, 1 to 2 minutes. Top with basil.

Calories: 180, fat: 5 g, saturated fat: 2 g, sodium: 290 mg, carbohydrate: 27 g, protein: 6 g.

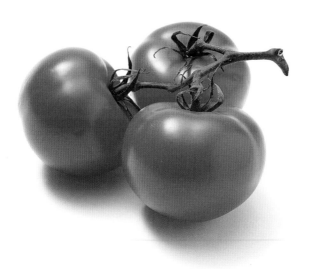

Grilled Halibut Steaks with Tomato & Red Pepper Salsa

Fish steaks make healthy fast food. In 20 minutes you can have a good supply of omega-3 fatty acids from the fish and vitamins C, B₆, and E as well as folate from the salsa.

PREPARATION TIME: 15 MINUTES

COOKING TIME: 4-6 MINUTES • SERVES 4

4 small halibut steaks
3 tbsp (45 mL) extra-virgin olive oil
Juice of 1 small orange
1 garlic clove, crushed

For salsa:
½ lb (250 g) plum tomatoes, diced
½ red bell pepper, seeded and diced
½ red onion, chopped fine
Juice of 1 small orange
¼ cup (50 mL) chopped fresh basil
1 tbsp (15 mL) balsamic vinegar
1 tsp (5 mL) sugar
Orange slices for garnish

1. Place halibut steaks in shallow baking dish. In small bowl, stir oil, orange juice, garlic, and salt and pepper to taste. Spoon over fish.

2. In serving bowl, combine the salsa ingredients with salt and pepper to taste and let stand at room temperature.

3. Heat lightly-oiled ridged cast-iron grill pan or heavy-based frying pan over high heat. Cook fish steaks for 2–3 minutes on each side, basting occasionally with oil mixture, until fish just flakes.

4. Serve fish with salsa.

Calories: 270, fat: 13 g, saturated fat: 2 g, sodium: 70 mg, carbohydrate: 11 g, protein: 25 g.

Asian Stuffed Shrimp Salad

Shrimp is a rich source of omega-3 fatty acids; the vegetables add vitamin C and folate.

PREPARATION TIME: 30 MINUTES

COOKING TIME: 10 MINUTES • SERVES 4

16 jumbo shrimp (1½ lb/750 g), peeled and deveined
⅓ cup (75 mL) chopped cilantro
1 clove garlic, minced
1 tbsp (15 mL) olive oil
2 carrots, julienned
2 scallions, cut into 2 x ¼-in (0.6-cm) strips
1 tbsp (15 mL) minced fresh ginger
2 tbsp (25 mL) lower-sodium soy sauce
2 tbsp (25 mL) chili sauce
4 tsp (20 mL) lime juice
1 tsp (5 mL) sugar
6 cups (1.5 L) torn romaine lettuce leaves
1 cucumber, peeled, halved lengthwise, seeded and sliced
2 tbsp (25 mL) chopped fresh mint

1. With paring knife, cut along back of shrimp until you have cut almost, but not quite through, to other side. In large bowl, toss together shrimp, cilantro, garlic and 1 tsp (15 mL) of oil; set aside.

2. In large nonstick skillet, heat remaining 2 tsp (10 mL) oil over moderate heat. Add carrots and scallions, and sauté for 2 minutes. Add ginger and cook for 2 minutes. Cool vegetable mixture to room temperature.

3. Preheat broiler. Place shrimp, cut side up, on broiler pan, pressing down to flatten shrimp slightly. Spoon vegetable mixture onto shrimp and broil 6 inches (15 cm) from heat for 4 minutes or until shrimp are just cooked through.

4. Meanwhile, in large bowl, combine soy sauce, chili sauce, lime juice and sugar. Add lettuce, cucumber and mint, tossing to combine. Serve shrimp on bed of the salad mixture.

Calories: 240, fat: 6 g, saturated fat: 1 g, sodium: 680 mg, carbohydrate: 9 g, protein: 38 g.

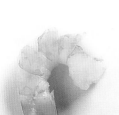

French Shrimp Stew

Seafood stews from the Mediterranean basin are frequently accented with the licorice-like taste of fennel, a prime source of vitamin C. In this aromatic dish, you will also get omega-3 fatty acids from the shrimp and more vitamin C from the tomatoes, peppers and onions, as well as some folate and vitamins E and B₆.

PREPARATION TIME: 30 MINUTES

COOKING TIME: 35 MINUTES • SERVES 4

- 1 red bell pepper, cut lengthwise into flat panels
- ½ tsp (2 mL) hot pepper sauce
- 1 tbsp (15 mL) olive oil
- 1 small onion, finely chopped
- 2 cloves garlic, minced
- 1 small bulb fennel, trimmed and cut into ½-in. (1-cm) pieces
- ⅔ cup (150 mL) canned no-salt-added tomatoes, chopped with their juice
- ½ cup (125 mL) chicken broth
- ¾ tsp (4 mL) grated orange zest
- ½ tsp (2 mL) salt
- 1 lb (500 g) medium shrimp, peeled and deveined
- 4 slices French or Italian bread, toasted

1. Preheat broiler. Place bell pepper pieces, skin side up, on broiler rack and broil 4 in. (10 cm) from heat 12 minutes or until skin is blackened. Place in paper bag to cool and then peel and transfer to a food processor or blender. Add hot pepper sauce and 1 tsp (15 mL) oil, and purée.

2. Meanwhile, in large nonstick skillet, heat remaining 2 tsp (10 mL) oil over moderate heat. Add onion and garlic, and sauté 5 minutes or until soft. Add fennel, and cook 7 minutes or until tender. Stir in tomatoes, broth, orange zest and salt. Bring to boil, reduce to a simmer, cover, and cook for 5 minutes.

3. Add shrimp to skillet and cook 4 minutes or until just cooked through. Stir roasted pepper purée into skillet. Serve stew with toast.

Calories: 220, fat: 5 g, saturated fat: 1 g, sodium: 730 mg, carbohydrate: 15 g, protein: 26 g.

Broiled Salmon With Avocado-Mango Salsa

If you like, make a small amount of lemon vinaigrette and toss with the lettuce before placing the salmon and salsa on top.

PREPARATION TIME: 10 MINUTES

COOKING TIME: 5 MINUTES • SERVES 4

- 2½ tsp (12 mL) paprika
- 2 (10 mL) ground coriander
- ¾ tsp (4 mL) salt
- 4 skinless, boneless salmon fillets (about 170 g/6 oz each)
- 1 large mango, peeled and cut into ½-in. (1-cm) chunks (1½ cups/375 mL)
- 1 hass avocado, peeled and cut into ½ in. (1-cm) chunks
- 1 cup (250 mL) canned chickpeas, drained and rinsed
- ⅓ cup (75 mL) chopped cilantro
- 1 tsp (5 mL) grated lemon zest
- 2 tbsp (25 mL) fresh lemon juice
- 2 tsp (10 mL) olive oil
- 6 cups (1.5 L) mesclun or frisée lettuce, torn into bite-size pieces

1. In large bowl, stir paprika, coriander and salt. Measure out 2 tsp (10 mL) spice mixtue and sprinkle over salmon, rubbing it into fish. Place salon, skin-side down, in broiler pan.

2. To remaining spice mixture, add mango, avocado, chickpeas, cilantro, lemon zest, lemon juice, and oil; toss to combine.

3. Broil salmon 6 in. (15 cm) from heat 5 minutes for medium. Serve salmon and salsa on a bed of frisée lettuce.

Calories: 551, fat: 29 g, saturated fat: 5 g, sodium: 745 mg, carbohydrate: 35 g, protein: 42 g.

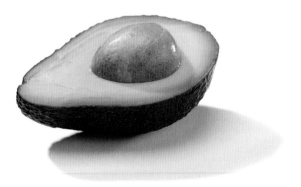

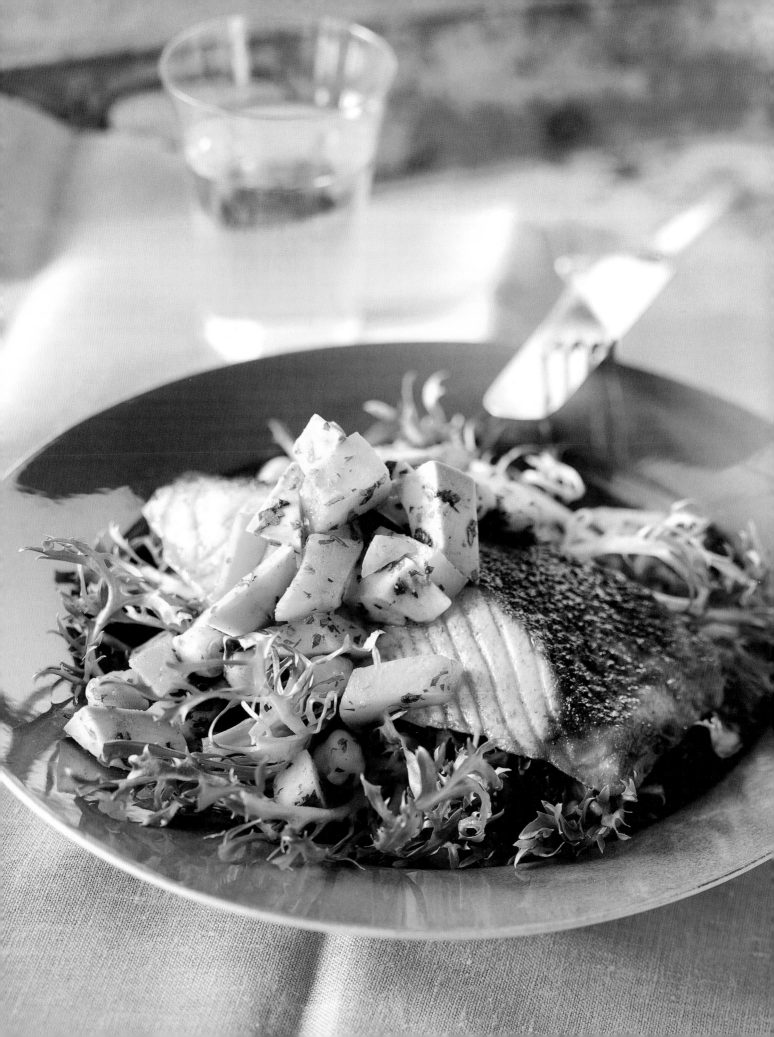

Penne with Sugar Snaps & Smoked Salmon

This is a pasta dish that gives you omega-3 fatty acids from the salmon, vitamin C from the lemon juice and zest, calcium and vitamin C from the sugar snap peas, and vitamin C and folate from the scallions.

PREPARATION TIME: 20 MINUTES

COOKING TIME: 15 MINUTES • SERVES 4

12 oz (375 g) penne or ziti pasta
1 lb (500 g) sugar snap peas, strings removed
1/3 cup (75 mL) snipped fresh dill
3 scallions, thinly sliced
3/4 cup (175 mL) chicken broth
3 tbsp (45 mL) reduced-fat sour cream
1 tbsp (15 mL) unsalted butter
1 tsp (5 mL) grated lemon zest
2 tbsp (25 mL) lemon juice
1/2 tsp (2 mL) salt
4 oz (125 g) smoked salmon, slivered

1. In large pot of boiling water, cook pasta according to package directions until firm-tender. Add sugar snaps to water during final minute of cooking; drain.

2. Meanwhile, in large bowl, combine dill, scallions, broth, sour cream, butter, lemon zest, lemon juice and salt. Add hot pasta and sugar snaps, tossing well. Add smoked salmon and toss again.

Calories: 450, fat: 7 g, saturated fat: 4 g, sodium: 850 mg, carbohydrate: 75 g, protein: 21 g.

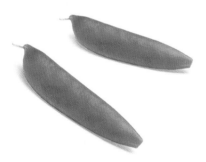

Creole-Style Beans

Robust beans, a prime source of folate, are cooked with the traditional Creole trinity of celery, onion and green pepper, offering up vitamins C, B₆, and more folate. The tomatoes give the dish vitamins C and E.

PREPARATION TIME: 10 MINUTES PLUS OVERNIGHT

SOAKING • COOKING TIME: 1 HOUR 15 MINUTES •

SERVES 4

3/4 cup (175 mL) dried cannellini or navy beans
1 tsp (5 mL) olive oil
3/4 cup (175 mL) vegetable broth
1 small fresh red chili pepper, seeded and finely chopped
1 garlic clove, minced
3 celery stalks, chopped
1/3 cup (75 mL) chopped onion
1 green bell pepper, seeded and chopped
1 tsp (5 mL) paprika
1 bay leaf
1 can (14 oz/398 mL) diced tomatoes

1. In medium bowl, combine beans and enough water to cover by 2 in. (5 cm), and let soak, chilled in refrigerator, overnight.

2. Drain beans in colander, and rinse well under cold water. In large pot, combine beans with enough water to cover. Boil rapidly for 15 minutes, skimming surface as necessary. Drain, rinse well and set aside.

3. Add oil, 1 tbsp (15 mL) broth, pepper flakes, garlic, celery, onion and green pepper to pot. Cook mixture, covered, over medium heat, shaking pan occasionally until vegetables have softened, about 10 minutes. Stir in paprika and cook, stirring, 1 minute. Add bay leaf, boiled beans, remaining broth and tomatoes and simmer, covered, until beans are tender, about 45 minutes, removing lid for last 10 minutes so that juices reduce. Season with salt and pepper to taste.

Calories: 100, fat: 2 g, saturated fat: 0 g, sodium: 125 mg, carbohydrate: 18 g, protein: 5 g.

Risotto with Spring Vegetables

This wholesome risotto is packed with fresh vegetables, which offer vitamins B₆, C, E and folate from the asparagus, vitamin C and folate from the beans, vitamin C and calcium from the peas, vitamin C and folate from the leek, not to mention even more calcium from the cheese.

PREPARATION TIME: 20 MINUTES PLUS 5 MINUTES

STANDING • COOKING TIME: 40-45 MINUTES •

SERVES 4

4 cups (1 L) vegetable broth
¼ tsp (1 mL) crumbled saffron threads
2 tbsp (25 mL) olive oil
3 carrots, chopped
2 garlic cloves, crushed
½ cup (125 mL) chopped well-washed leek
½ lb (250 g) Arborio rice
¼ lb (125 g) asparagus spears (about 8), cut into 1-in. (2.5 cm) lengths
¼ lb (125 g) green beans, cut into 1-in. (2.5-cm) lengths
¾ cup (175 mL) green peas, defrosted if frozen
¼ cup (50 mL) chopped fresh herbs, such as chives, dill, flat-leaved parsley and tarragon
½ cup (125 mL) grated Parmesan cheese

1. In pot, warm broth, then add saffron and let stand off heat for 10 minutes.

2. Meanwhile, in large skillet, heat oil over medium-low heat, add carrots, garlic and leek and cook, stirring, until softened, about 10 minutes. Add rice to vegetables and stir 1 minute or until grains are glossy.

3. Return broth to heat and simmer. Add one ladleful of broth to rice, stirring continuously until absorbed. Continue adding broth, a ladleful at a time, and stirring for 15 minutes.

4. Add asparagus, beans and peas to rice and continue stirring and adding stock until rice and vegetables are tender. (This should take 15–20 minutes). Remove pot from heat, stir in herbs and Parmesan, and let rest, covered, 5 minutes. Season with salt and pepper to taste.

Calories: 390, fat: 13 g, saturated fat: 4 g, sodium: 240 mg, carbohydrate: 58 g, protein: 15 g.

Tex-Mex Turkey, Corn & Barley Casserole

Barley gives you vitamin B₆ and folate, among other good things. You get even more B₆ from the turkey and peppers in this hearty dish.

PREPARATION TIME: 10-12 MINUTES

COOKING TIME: 1 HOUR 15 MINUTES • SERVES 4

2 tbsp (25 mL) canola oil
2 onions, coarsely chopped
1 large red or green bell pepper, coarsely chopped
1 tsp (5 mL) finely chopped hot chili pepper
1 cup (250 mL) pearl barley, sorted and rinsed
1¾ cups (425 mL) chicken broth
1 can (14 oz/398 mL) crushed tomatoes
⅛ tsp (0.5 mL) each salt and pepper
2 cups (500 mL) shredded cooked turkey
1 cup (250 mL) frozen corn kernels, thawed

1. Preheat oven to 325°F (160°C). In flameproof casserole, heat oil over moderate heat. Sauté onions, bell pepper and chili pepper, stirring, 7 minutes or until softened and lightly browned.

2. Add barley and cook, stirring, until well coated with oil. Pour in chicken broth and crushed tomatoes, and season with salt and pepper.

3. Bring to boil, then stir in turkey. Cover casserole and cook in oven, stirring occasionally, 55 minutes or until almost all liquid has been absorbed and barley is nearly tender.

4. Stir in corn kernels, cover casserole, and cook 5 to 10 minutes longer, until heated through.

Calories: 475, fat: 9 g, saturated fat: 2 g, sodium: 262 mg, carbohydrate: 65 g, protein: 31 g.

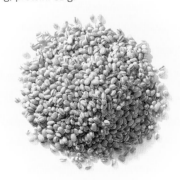

Herbed Polenta

The milk and cheese in this recipe give you calcium; the cornmeal provides some vitamin B$_6$.

PREPARATION TIME: 5 MINUTES PLUS CHILLING TIME

COOKING TIME: 25 MINUTES • SERVES 6

1 cup (250 mL) yellow cornmeal
2 cups (500 mL) 1% milk
⅛ tsp (0.5 mL) each salt and pepper
2 tbsp (25 mL) chopped parsley or basil
2 tbsp (25 mL) finely grated Parmesan
   cheese

1. Combine cornmeal with 1 cup (250 mL) water in small bowl. In nonstick pot, bring milk and 1 cup (250 mL) water to a boil. Season with salt and pepper.

2. Reduce heat slightly and slowly stir cornmeal into milk mixture. Cook, stirring constantly, about 5 minutes or until mixture boils and thickens slightly.

3. Reduce heat to very low and simmer polenta gently, stirring frequently, 10 minutes or until mixture is smooth and thickened.

4. Remove pot from heat. Add chopped herbs and cheese and stir well to mix thoroughly.

5. Turn polenta out onto nonstick baking pan and spread to depth of ¼ in. (0.5 cm) with a palette knife. Chill 2 hours to set. Preheat broiler.

6. With cookie cutter, cut rounds from polenta. Use trimmings to make more. Or cut into 6 wedges. Broil on rack about 5 minutes, until golden.

Calories: 128, fat: 2 g, saturated fat: 1 g, sodium: 128 mg, carbohydrate: 22 g, protein: 6 g.

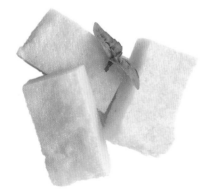

Apricot-Maple Acorn Squash

Acorn squash, with its bright orange flesh, gives you lots of vitamin C and vitamin B$_6$. With maple syrup and apricot jam, it's delectable.

PREPARATION TIME: 5 MINUTES • COOKING TIME:

1 HOUR OR UNTIL IT'S TENDER • SERVES 4

2 one-pound (500-g) acorn squashes
¼ cup (50 mL) apricot jam
2 tbsp (25 mL) maple syrup

1. Halve and seed squashes.

2. Place in baking pan, cut sides down, add ⅓ cup (75 mL) water, cover with foil, and bake for 25 minutes at 400°F (200°C). Drain. Turn cut sides up.

3. Stir together apricot jam and maple syrup. Spoon into squash. Bake 35 minutes or until tender.

Calories: 170, fat: 0 g, saturated fat: 0 g, sodium: 15 mg, carbohydrate: 43 g, protein: 2 g.

Orange-Glazed Carrots

This is a way to make your vitamin C—from carrots and oranges—irresistible.

PREPARATION TIME: 5 MINUTES

COOKING TIME: 15 MINUTES • SERVES 4

1 lb (500 g) very small, peeled carrots
   (or pre-peeled "baby" carrots)
¼ cup (50 mL) orange juice
2 tbsp (25 mL) orange marmalade
   (or apricot jam)
2 tsp (10 mL) unsalted butter
½ tsp (2 mL) salt

1. In pot with a steamer insert, cook carrots over water until crisp-tender.

2. In large skillet, heat orange juice, marmalade jam, butter and salt.

3. Add carrots and cook over moderate heat until nicely glazed.

Calories: 90, fat: 3 g, saturated fat: 2 g, sodium: 280 mg, carbohydrate: 17 g, protein: 1 g.

Roasted New Potatoes

New potatoes, full of vitamins C and B$_6$, appear in the late spring or early summer. Enjoy!

PREPARATION TIME: 10 MINUTES

COOKING TIME: 45 MINUTES • SERVES 8

1½ lb (750 g) small new potatoes, scrubbed
3 cloves garlic, thinly sliced
2 tbsp (25 mL) olive or canola oil
½ tsp (2 mL) crumbled rosemary

1. Preheat oven to 400°F (200°C). In large bowl, combine potatoes with garlic, oil and rosemary.

2. Transfer to roasting pan, arranging in one layer, and roast 45 minutes or until golden and cooked through.

Calories: 219, fat: 8 g, saturated fat: 1 g, sodium: 16 mg, carbohydrate: 35 g, protein: 3 g.

Sweet Roasted Squash with Shallots

Roasted vegetables are sweetened with a touch of maple syrup. It's a lovely way to get your vitamin C and folate from both the shallots and the squash.

PREPARATION TIME: 15 MINUTES

COOKING TIME: 30-35 MINUTES • SERVES 4

2 lb (1 kg) butternut squash
8 shallots, peeled
3 sprigs fresh thyme
1 tsp (5 mL) olive oil
2 tsp (10 mL) pure maple syrup

1. Preheat oven to 375°F (190°C). Halve squash lengthwise, scrape out seeds, and remove peel with a vegetable peeler. Cut into 1¼-in (0.6-cm) cubes.

2. Combine squash, shallots, thyme, oil, syrup, and salt and pepper to taste in roasting pan and toss to coat vegetables. Roast vegetables until tender and golden brown, 30–35 minutes, turning occasionally.

Calories: 120, fat: 2 g, saturated fat: 0 g, sodium: 10 mg, carbohydrate: 29 g, protein: 2 g.

Sweet Potato & Apple Bake

Unlike the familiar marshmallow topping, apples make a substantial nutritional contribution to a sweet-potato casserole, which abounds in vitamin C from the sweet potatoes, apples, onion and lemon juice, plus B$_6$ from the sweet potatoes.

PREPARATION TIME: 20 MINUTES

COOKING TIME: 45 MINUTES • SERVES 4

1 tbsp (15 mL) unsalted butter
1 onion, finely chopped
2 lb (1 kg) sweet potatoes, peeled and thinly sliced
2 McIntosh apples, cut into ½-in. (1-cm) thick wedges
3 tbsp (45 mL) sugar
2 tbsp (25 mL) lemon juice
¾ cup (175 mL) chicken broth
½ tsp (2 mL) salt
¼ tsp (1 mL) pepper

1. Preheat oven to 450°F (230°C). In very large nonstick skillet, heat butter over moderate heat. Add onion and sauté 5 minutes or until tender.

2. Add sweet potatoes, apples, 2 tbsp (25 mL) sugar and lemon juice, and cook until sugar has melted. Add broth, salt, and pepper, and bring to boil.

3. Transfer mixture to 7-in. x 11-in. (18-cm x 28-cm) glass baking dish. Cover with foil and bake for 25 minutes or until sweet potatoes are tender. Uncover, sprinkle with remaining 1 tbsp (15 mL) sugar, and bake 10 minutes or until lightly browned.

Calories: 350, fat: 4 g, saturated fat: 2 g, sodium: 290 mg, carbohydrate: 76 g, protein: 5 g.

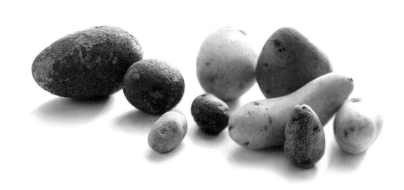

Pineapple Foster

Bananas Foster is a beloved New Orleans dessert, created in the 1950s at Brennan's Restaurant. This pineapple variation, in which the fruit is a good source of vitamin C, will bring raves. The frozen yogourt adds calcium as well as a cool taste contrast.

PREPARATION TIME: 15 MINUTES

COOKING TIME: 10 MINUTES • SERVES 4

4 tsp (20 mL) unsalted butter
3 tbsp (45 mL) packed light brown sugar
¼ tsp (1 mL) ground nutmeg
6 slices (¾-in./1.75-cm thick) fresh
   pineapple, cored and cut into quarters
3 tbsp (45 mL) dark rum
2 tbsp (25 mL) Grand Marnier, or other
   orange liqueur
1⅓ cup (325 mL) vanilla frozen yogourt

1. In a large skillet, melt butter over moderate heat. When it begins to foam, add brown sugar and nutmeg, and heat until sugar has melted. Add pineapple and cook, tossing often, 4 minutes or until pineapple is warmed through.

2. Remove pan from heat, sprinkle rum and Grand Marnier over pineapple, and ignite alcohol with a long match. Return pan to heat and shake until alcohol burns off.

3. Serve pineapple slices and sauce with the frozen yogourt.

Calories: 280, fat: 5 g, saturated fat: 3 g,
sodium: 35 mg, carbohydrate: 48 g,
protein: 5 g.

Caramelized Orange Compote

Oranges are a prime source of vitamin C; here's a way to dress them up.

PREPARATION TIME: 10 MINUTES

COOKING TIME: 2 MINUTES • SERVES 4

4 peeled and segmented navel oranges
¼ cup (50 mL) brown sugar
¼ tsp (1 mL) cinnamon
1 tbsp (15 mL) slivered orange zest

1. Preheat broiler. Place peeled and segmented navel oranges in gratin dish or shallow broiler-proof baking dish.

2. Sprinkle with brown sugar, cinnamon and zest. Broil 2 minutes or until sugar melts.

Calories: 120, fat: 0 g, saturated fat: 0 g, sodium: 5 mg,
carbohydrate: 30 g, protein: 1 g.

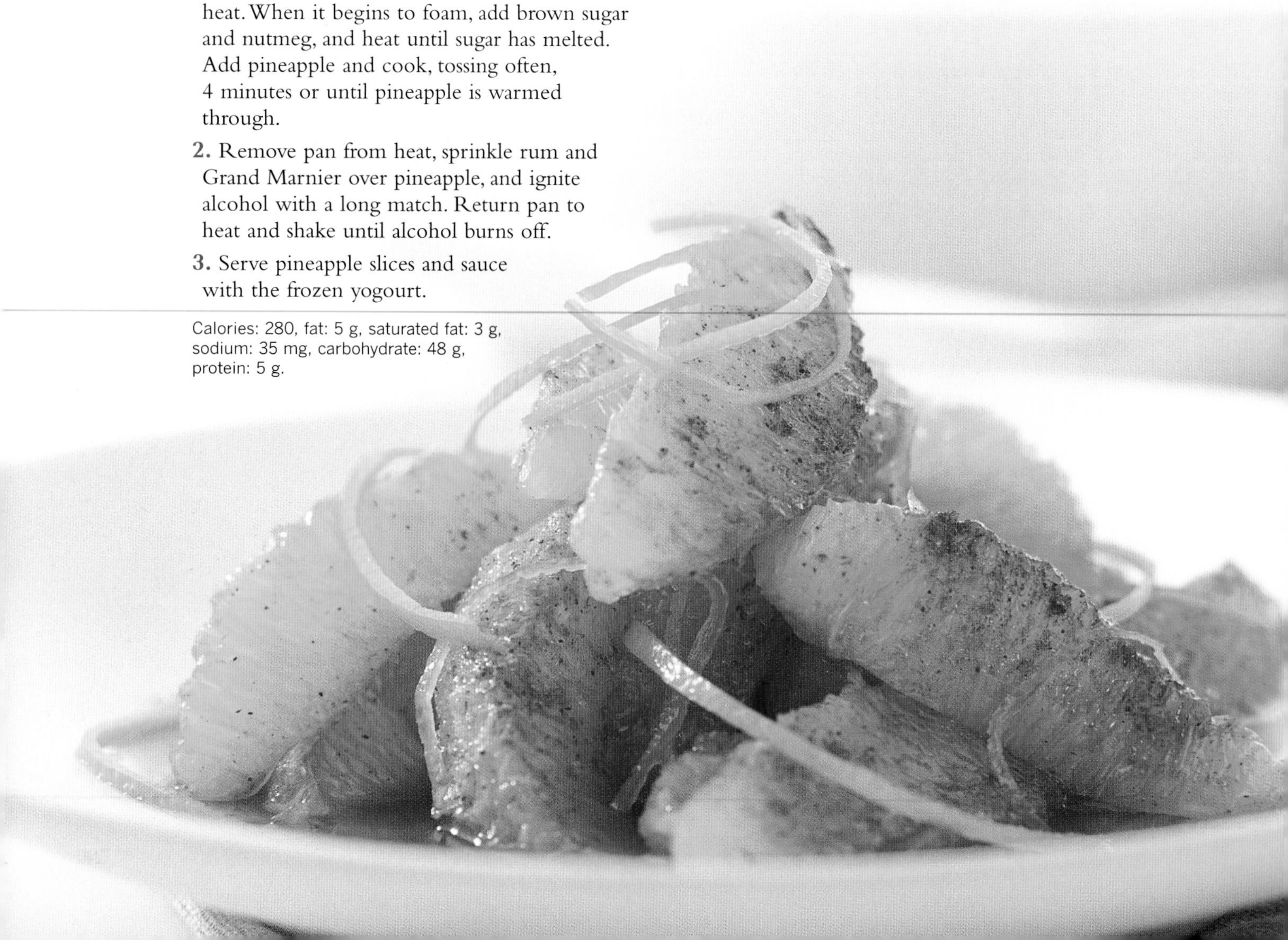

Berry Sorbet

Sorbets, made only from fruit and sweetener—no milk—are fat and cholesterol free. You'll always have room for a dessert as light and refreshing as this one, particularly when it is packed with vitamin C from lime juice and both kinds of berries.

PREPARATION TIME: 8 MINUTES

COOKING TIME: 5 MINUTES • FREEZING TIME: 5 HOURS

MAKES SIX ½ CUP SERVINGS

½ cup (125 mL) lime juice
2 tbsp (25 mL) grenadine syrup or 2 tbsp
(25 mL) water plus 1 tbsp (15 mL) sugar
⅓ cup (75 mL) water
1 package (12 oz/375 g) frozen unsweetened
raspberries, thawed
1 package (12 oz/375 g) frozen unsweetened
strawberries, thawed

1. In medium pot, bring lime juice, sugar, grenadine and water to boil over moderate heat. Cook 1 minute or until sugar is dissolved.

2. In food processor or blender, whirl raspberries and strawberries 30 seconds or until puréed. Press fruit through fine sieve to eliminate seeds. You should have 2 cups (500 mL) purée; if not, add enough water to make up the difference.

3. Stir purée into sugar syrup. Transfer mixture to an 8-in. x 8-in. x 2-in. (20-cm x 20-cm x 5-cm) pan, cover with plastic wrap, and freeze 2 hours or until the centre is almost frozen. Remove sorbet from freezer and beat until smooth. Return to freezer for 45 minutes, then beat again until smooth. Freeze 2 to 3 hours more before serving.

Calories: 125, fat: 0 g, saturated fat: 0 g, sodium: 1 mg, carbohydrate: 33 g, protein: 1 g.

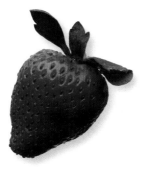

Chocolate-Hazelnut Cheesecake

Toasted hazelnuts top this velvety tofu and cottage cheese (major sources of calcium) cheesecake. The egg offers vitamin D; the canola oil, omega-3 fatty acids.

PREPARATION TIME: 15 MINUTES • COOKING TIME:

50 MINUTES • CHILLING TIME: 2 HOURS • SERVES 12

⅓ cup (75 mL) hazelnuts
1 cup (250 mL) graham cracker crumbs
(5 oz/150 g)
1 tbsp (15 mL) canola oil
¼ cup (50 mL) unsweetened cocoa powder
1 lb (500 g) silken tofu
1 cup (250 mL) creamed (4%) cottage cheese
1 oz (30 g) semisweet chocolate, melted
½ cup (125 mL) granulated sugar
⅔ cup (150 mL) packed light brown sugar
2 tbsp (25 mL) flour
1 egg
2 egg whites
1 tsp (5 mL) vanilla extract

1. Preheat oven to 375°F (190°C). Toast hazelnuts on baking sheet 7 minutes or until skins begin to crinkle (leave the oven on). Transfer hazelnuts to kitchen towel and rub to remove skin (some will remain). When hazelnuts are cool enough to handle, coarsely chop and set aside.

2. In small bowl, stir crumbs, oil and 1 tbsp (15 mL) water. Press mixture into bottom and partway up sides of 9½-in. (24-cm) springform pan. Bake 8 minutes, until crust is set. Cool on rack. Reduce oven temperature to 350°F (180°C).

3. In small bowl, combine cocoa and ¼ cup (50 mL) water. In food processor, combine tofu, cottage cheese, melted semisweet chocolate, granulated sugar, brown sugar, flour, whole egg, egg whites, vanilla and cocoa mixture, and process until smooth.

4. Pour batter into prepared crust and bake 40 minutes. Reduce oven temperature to 250°F (120°C), sprinkle nuts on top, and bake 10 minutes or until cheesecake is just set. Cool to room temperature; refrigerate for 2 hours or until chilled.

Calories: 210, fat: 7 g, saturated fat: 2 g, sodium: 190 mg, carbohydrate: 30 g, protein: 8 g.

Three Berry Fool

Although many recipes call for straining out the seeds from raspberry purées and sauces, we have purposely left them in because the seeds account for a good amount of the dietary fibre.

PREPARATION TIME: 15 MINUTES

STANDING TIME: 4 HOURS

COOKING TIME: 6 MINUTES • SERVES 4

1 qt (1 L) plain low-fat yogourt
1 package (12 oz/375 g) frozen unsweetened
    rapsberries, thawed
2 cups (500 mL) frozen unsweetened
    strawberries, thawed
½ cup (125 mL) sugar
1½ tsp (7 mL) vanilla extract
3 tsp (15 mL) cornstarch blended with
    2 tbsp (25 mL) water
1 package (12 oz/375 g) frozen unsweetened
    blueberries
2 tbsp (25 mL) orange juice
¼ tsp (1 mL) pepper
¼ tsp (1 mL) allspice
1 tbsp (15 mL) fresh lemon juice

1. Spoon yogourt into fine-mesh strainer set over bowl. Let stand 4 hours at room temperature.

2. In food processor, purée raspberries, strawberries, ¼ cup (50 mL) sugar and ½ tsp (2 mL) vanilla. Transfer to small pot and boil over medium heat. Stir in ½ cornstarch mixture and boil, stirring, 1 minute, until lightly thickened. Let cool, cover, and refrigerate.

3. In small pot, combine blueberries, orange juice, pepper, allspice and 2 tbsp (25 mL) sugar; simmer. Cook, stirring frequently 5 minutes, or until blueberries are tender. Stir in remaining cornstarch mixture and boil; cook, stirring constantly, 1 minute, or until thickened. Transfer to bowl and stir in lemon juice; cover and refrigerate.

4. In medium bowl, combine the drained yogourt, remaining sugar and remaining vanilla.

5. Spoon berry mixture into 4 bowls. Spoon blueberry mixture into centres and top with yogourt. Gently swirl mixture to lightly marble the yogourt with fruit purée.

Calories: 331, fat: 4.5 g, saturated fat: 0.8 g, sodium: 0 mg, carbohydrate: 33 g, protein: 13 g.

Ginger Pancake with Banana-Walnut Topping

Serve this oversized pancake for dessert or as the main attraction at a Sunday brunch.

PREPARATION TIME: 10 MINUTES

COOKING TIME: 20 MINUTES • SERVES 4

½ cup (75 mL) walnuts
½ cup (125 mL) flour
½ cup (125 mL) 1% milk
1 large egg
1 large egg white
1 tbsp (15 mL) light olive oil
1 tbsp (15 mL) butter, melted
2 tbsp (25 mL) granulated sugar
1 (5 mL) vanilla extract
¼ (1 mL) salt
⅓ cup (75 mL) finely chopped crystallized
    ginger
¼ cup (50 mL) fresh lime juice
2 tbsp (25 mL) packed light brown sugar
3 bananas, thinly sliced

1. Preheat oven to 350°F (180°C). Toast walnuts 5 minutes, or until crisp and fragrant. When walnuts are cool enough to handle, coarsely chop.

2. Increase oven temperature to 425°F (220°C). Lightly oil nonstick skillet and place in oven.

3. In large bowl, stir together flour, milk, whole egg, egg white, oil, butter, granulated sugar, vanilla and salt until well combined. Stir in ginger.

4. Pour batter into hot pan, return pan to oven, and bake 12 to 15 minutes, or until pancake has puffed and is golden brown.

5. Meanwhile, in large skillet, combine lime juice and brown sugar, and cook over medium heat until sugar has melted. Add sliced bananas and cook 3 minutes, or until bananas have softened. Stir in walnuts.

6. To serve, cut pancake into wedges and top with banana-walnut mixture.

Calories: 402, fat: 15 g, saturated fat: 3.6 g, sodium: 35 mg, carbohydrate: 63 g, protein: 7 g.

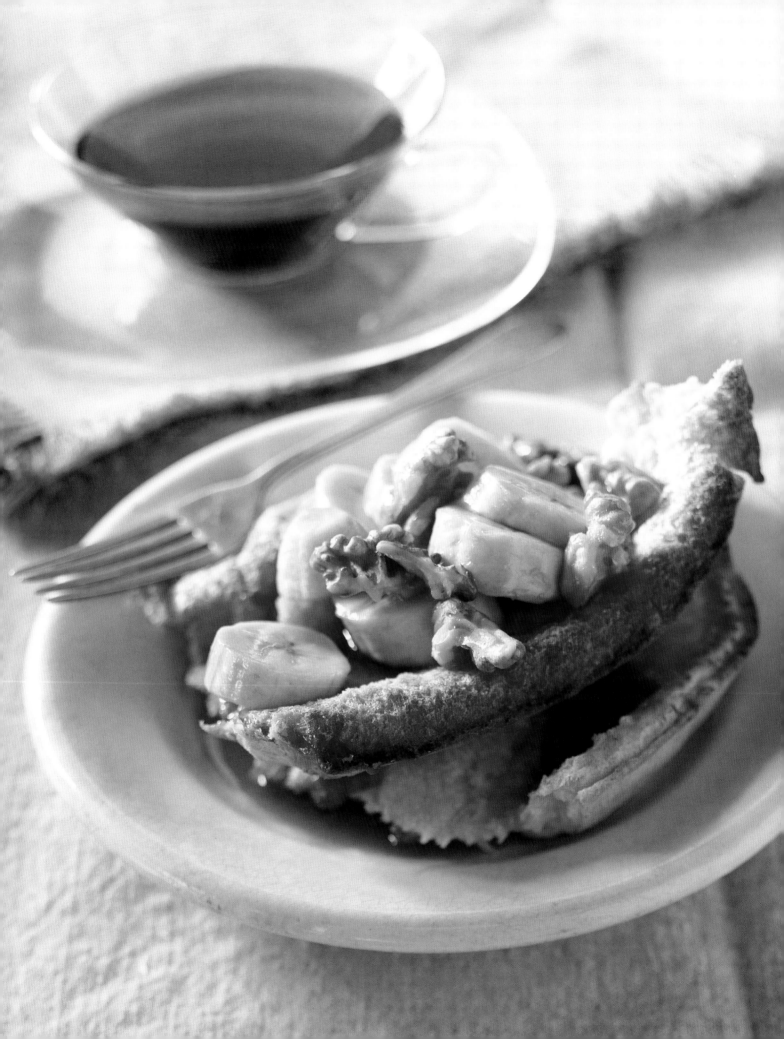

Mixed Berry Tart

Sweet berries and flaky crust add up to an irresistible dessert rich in antioxidants and fibre. Use a blend of berries or just one type. Vary the flavours with lime juice instead of lemon juice and ginger instead of cinnamon.

PREPARATION TIME: 2 HOURS, 20 MINUTES

COOKING TIME: 40 MINUTES • SERVES 12

¼ cup (50 mL) ice water, without ice
3 tbsp (45 mL) low-fat plain yogourt
1 cup (250 mL) whole-grain pastry flour
½ cup (125 mL) all-purpose flour
1 tbsp (15 mL) + ⅓ cup (75 mL) sugar
¼ tsp (1 mL) ground cinnamon
¼ tsp (1 mL) salt
7 tbsp (105 mL) margarine or butter
5 cups (1.25 L) mixed berries, such as blueberries, raspberries, and strawberries
2 tbsp (25 mL) cornstarch
1 tbsp (15 mL) lemon juice
Icing sugar (optional)

1. In measuring cup, whisk together water and yogourt. In food processor, combine pastry and all-purpose flour, 1 tbsp (15 mL) sugar, cinnamon and salt. Add margarine and pulse until mixture resembles coarse crumbs. With motor running, gradually add yogourt mixture and process just until ingredients come together. Gather dough into ball. Wrap in plastic and refrigerate 2 hours.

2. Preheat oven to 350°F (180°C). In large bowl, combine berries, cornstarch, lemon juice, and ⅓ cup (75 mL) sugar and toss gently.

3. Shape dough into 6 small balls. Roll out each ball on lightly floured work surface to about a 6-in. (15-cm) circle. Using six 4-in. (10-cm) tartlet pans with removable bottoms, line pans with dough. Evenly distribute fruit mixture into pans.

4. Bake until filling is bubbling and crust is browned, 15 to 20 minutes. Transfer to rack 15 minutes. Remove from pans and cool completely. Each tartlet is 2 servings. Dust with icing sugar.

Calories: 165, fat: 3 g, saturated fat: 0 g, sodium: 128 mg, carbohydrate: 3 g, protein: 3 g.

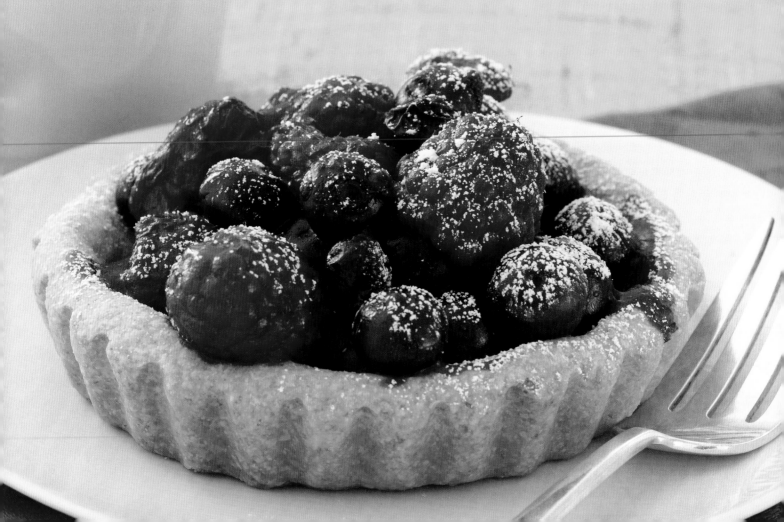